SUCCESSFUL GRANT WRITING

Strategies for Health and Human Service Professionals

Second Edition

Laura N. Gitlin, PhD is Professor in the Department of Occupational Therapy and founding Director of the Community and Homecare Research Division (CHORD) at Jefferson College of Health Professions, Thomas Jefferson University. Chord's mission is to develop and test innovative behavioral and environmental approaches to helping older people with physical frailty remain at home, supporting family caregivers, and enhancing life quality of persons with dementia. Dr. Gitlin is a nationally and internationally recognized and well funded researcher, having received research and training grants from both federal agencies and private foundations, including the Alzheimer's Association and the National Institutes of Health. She currently has over $6 million of committed research grant monies and has helped garner close to $20 million in grant funding over the past 20 years. As part of a current Geriatric Leadership Award funded by the National Institute on Aging, she is establishing an infrastructure for funded aging research at Thomas Jefferson University. Dr. Gitlin has also served as a grant reviewer for the National Institute on Disability and Rehabilitation Research, the Alzheimer's Association, the National Institute on Aging, the Agency for Health Research and Quality, and the American Occupational Therapy Foundation. She has published extensively in peer-reviewed journals, is a co-author of a research text on quantitative and qualitative research methodologies, and has two books forthcoming.

Dr. Kevin J. Lyons, PhD is Associate Dean in the College of Health Professions and the College of Graduate Studies and Director of the Center for Collaborative Research at Thomas Jefferson University. He has over 25 years of experience in higher education as a faculty member and administrator. He has served on the Institute of Medicine of the National Academy of Sciences' Committee on Health Services Research: Training and Workforce Issues, has written a white paper for the National Commission on Allied Health. In addition, he is Editor of the *Journal of Allied Health*: the scholarly journal of the Association of Schools of Allied Health Professions, and has received the J. Warren Perry Distinguished Author Award and been elected a Fellow in that organization. Dr. Lyons has presented numerous papers at national and international scientific meetings and has been a frequent consultant to universities and government agencies on issues such as research development and program improvement and has received significant funding from the Bureau of Health Professions to conduct research institutes to advance the research mission of the allied health and chiropractic professions. Dr. Lyons has served on peer review panels for FIPSE, OSERS and NIDRR in the U.S. Department of Education, the Bureau of Health Professions and for numerous professional journals.

SUCCESSFUL GRANT WRITING

*Strategies for Health and
Human Service Professionals*

Second Edition

Laura N. Gitlin, PhD
Kevin J. Lyons, PhD

 Springer Publishing Company

DEDICATION

To Eduardo, Keith, and Eric,
Siempre.
El camino de mi vida.

LNG

As before, to Brendan, Margaret, Patrick and Bridget with
love. And to the newest additions: Matt, Christine, Mike,
Lauren and especially the next generation of grantwriters,
Ryan, Ashley and Madison. For you it's worthwhile.

KJL

To our students and colleagues and to all new
investigators whose creative ideas and dedication
to the improvement of health and health care delivery
for all makes grantsmanship a most worthy endeavor.

Springer Publishing Company, Inc.
536 Broadway
New York, NY 10012-3955

Acquisitions Editor: Helvi Gold
Production Editor: Matt Fenton
Cover design by Joanne E. Honigman

04 05 06 07 08 / 5 4 3 2

Library of Congress Cataloging-in-Publication Data

Gitlin, Laura N., 1952–
    Successful grant writing : strategies for health and human service professionals /
Laura N. Gitlin, Kevin J. Lyons, authors.
        p. cm.
    Includes bibliographical references and index.
    ISBN 0-8261-9261-0
    1. Proposal writing in human services. 2. Medical care—Research grants. 3. Public
health—Research grants. 4. Proporal writing for grants. I. Lyons, Kevin J. II. Title.
HV41.2.G58   2004
361'.0068'1—dc22   2003063325

Printed in the United States of America by Integrated Book Technology

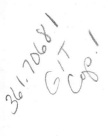

Contents

v

Preface

There are many books, pamphlets, and newsletters on writing competitive grant applications. Few, however, address the topic from the perspective of the health and human service professional. Fewer still focus on helping the novice develop proficiency in grant writing. *Successful Grant Writing: Strategies for Health and Human Services Professionals* is specially designed and written for these professionals in academic and practice settings who are either inexperienced grant writers or who have had some success, but would like to expand their knowledge and become more competent in obtaining external support.

The health and human service professions continue to be at a crossroad. They are transforming from occupations and redefining themselves as true professions. Obtaining external funding to examine professional issues, improve services, or develop and test new education, service, and research models is an essential activity of health professionals.

This book includes a range of strategies and work models that are appropriate for health and human service professionals, who have different growth needs and opportunities for funding than traditional research scientists. It is our hope that it will contribute to the transformation of health care by providing a framework for understanding the funding world and offering definitive and effective strategies for success in obtaining external support.

HOW TO USE THIS BOOK

After discussing the importance of developing a research career and obtaining a knowledge of the language and basic components of grantsmanship in Part I, this book moves the reader to developing his or her own ideas for funding in Part II, writing the sections of a proposal in Part III, organizing different types of project structures in Part IV, understanding the review process in Part V, and, finally, managing a grant award when it is received in Part VI. Each chapter describes a specific aspect of grantsmanship and suggests innovative strategies for implementing the information that is presented. These strategies may be beneficial to individuals or departments in academic, clinical, or community-based settings. They can be used by an individual to outline a course of action and pursue an independent grant funded program, or by a department to plan a systematic approach to capturing external funding. The appendices contain helpful materials, such as a list of key acronyms, examples of time lines, and sample budget sheets.

The guidelines and suggestions in this book are based on more than 20 years of experience by each of the authors in obtaining external support for education and research programs and working with individuals in the health and human service fields, as well as from interviews with experienced grant writers and program officers in key federal agencies and foundations.

Introduction

You have a great idea that you believe can significantly improve the educational program for your students or services for your clients. To carry out the idea you probably will require financial support. How can you obtain this support?

One way is to apply for a grant from the federal government, a private foundation, or a corporation. A grant is a mechanism by which an agency awards money to fund a research study or other activity, such as an educational program, service program, demonstration, or research project.

The task of writing a grant proposal, or even knowing how to get started, can be daunting, especially if it is your first attempt. As with any venture, grantsmanship has a language of its own, a set of rules, and relatively standard procedures, all of which you can learn and become successful in using.

But you may well ask why you need to learn the process of grantsmanship. After all, it involves considerable time and effort and requires a new set of skills. There is more than one purpose for obtaining a grant. Obviously, if you need money to develop and implement a new program, a grant is one way to obtain that support. However, there are other very important but less tangible reasons to pursue external funding.

What can grants do for you?

Grants can help you:

- Develop and advance scientific knowledge in your field.
- Support training and research activities.
- Provide support for institutional activities.

- Expand opportunities for educating students and clinicians.
- Legitimize your research program or training projects.
- Enhance the prestige of your institution.
- Advance your professional career.

Let's examine each of these reasons more closely.

Develop and advance scientific knowledge in your field: The basic mission of most federal funding agencies and the reason those in the health and human service professions pursue research or educational grants is to develop and advance knowledge in a particular field. For example, funding for a research study on the determinants of older women's compliance with mammography or examining the impact of a home intervention to help frail elders is critical for advancing knowledge in these areas and improving the health and functioning of individuals and groups. The support for model educational programs also leads to new and effective instructional methods that can improve the practice of health and human service professionals.

Support training and research activities: Another purpose of grant funding is to support the development and implementation of new training programs. Developing new programs can be expensive, and institutions are often hesitant to support new ventures unless they have been systematically tested and shown to be effective. Training or education grants can be important catalysts for implementing change in an institution's approach to educating health and human service professionals.

Provide support for institutional activities: Success in gaining external funding can also contribute to the vitality and financial health of your department, school, or agency. The direct costs derived from a funded project may support a special program your institution wants to run or, in some cases, contribute toward its general operating expenses. At a university, funds might pay for part of your salary or that of other important staff members, as well as statistical support or consultants, and expenses such as supplies and professional travel. The facilities and administrative (F&A) cost recovery, also referred to as indirect costs, a term defined later in this book, helps defray operating costs such as heat, light, and telephone use.

Expand opportunities for educating students and clinicians: As college tuition continues to rise, it becomes increasingly difficult for students to afford an education, particularly in the health and human service fields, where low salaries make it difficult to pay back loans for tuition. Many Ph.D. students in the basic biomedical sciences are often fully or partially supported by funded research projects. Similar opportunities are available in many of the health and human service fields, primarily through the support of positions such as research assistants, interviewers, or project coordinators.

Legitimize your research program or training projects: Obtaining funding for your project provides public recognition of the worth of your educational or research program. Grant applications are reviewed and approved by a jury of your peers, and this process provides external validation and legitimization of your work. An award indicates that experts in the field acknowledge your idea as important and worthy of public or private support.

Enhance the prestige of your institution: Health and human service professionals in higher education are increasingly encouraged to obtain external funding, not only to advance knowledge in their field but also to contribute to the prestige of their institution. External funding is often used as an index of the prestige of a college or university and the quality of its faculty. As a result, many universities measure quality, in part, by the extent to which faculty members obtain external funding. It is no longer true that schools or departments educating health and human service professionals will be recognized as contributing to the institution only through the training of competent clinicians. These schools are now evaluated on their contribution to the overall research mission of the university. In some cases, their continuation in the institution is dependent, in part, on the extent to which the research mission is successfully pursued.

Advance your professional career: A funded grant also enhances your professional standing, both within the institution and in the profession at large. Funded health professionals become known among their peers through professional newsletters, journals, or other national forums. Thus, funding success not only advances your knowledge base and professional development, but will also provide increased professional prestige and job mobility.

Part I

The Perspective of Funding Agencies

Welcome to the world of grantsmanship! Grantsmanship is the process of using knowledge and implementing a series of activities to obtain a grant to carry out a program. It is both an art and a technical skill that involves hard work, and sometimes trial and error prior to a successful outcome.

A basic tenet of grantsmanship is that being well informed about the process and the funding source is critical for success. The more you know about an agency and its funding priorities, the greater the likelihood that you will be able to write a proposal that is competitive and matches the intent of the funding source.

The funding environment is constantly changing. This is especially true today, in light of health care reform. Therefore, finding the right funder for your particular idea takes time and requires knowledge of multiple sources that provide information about funding opportunities. Therefore, we begin chapter 1 by describing the perspective of funding agencies and introducing the language they use. We then examine the sources of information about funding opportunities and help interpret their messages in chapter 2.

1

Chapter 1

Getting Started

- A Grant Story
- The Language of Grantsmanship
- A Research Career Trajectory

Do you have a great idea, but need money to carry it out? If you do, then who will pay for it? Where can you obtain information about sources for support? What is the best way to convince a funding source to support your idea?

These are questions that many health and human services professionals ask. Fortunately, there are agencies in both the public and private sectors who have money for worthy projects. Your job is to first find out where and how to look for these pockets of money and then to learn how to write a grant application that will convince a funding agency of your project's importance. This is the essence of grantsmanship.

The first point to understand about grantsmanship is that you are not competing with a funding agency. The purpose of federal funding agencies and private foundations is to give money away. Consider, for example, agencies of the federal government that are funded by Congress to solve problems facing the American people. Each agency is charged with the responsibility of addressing a different issue, such as women's health or cancer prevention. Based on their charge, the agency sets priorities for the types of research or educational grant programs to fund. Each year these agencies have to compete for funds from Congress to support their grant programs. To obtain congressional funds, an agency must demonstrate to Congress that significant progress is being made in addressing a problem area. Indices of progress include the number of grant proposals submitted to the agency, the quality of the grant programs that they have funded and the contributions that these programs have made to the advancement of knowledge and practice. Therefore, it is in an agency's best interest to encourage the submission and approval of as many good proposals as possible.

A second point to remember is that not every "great" idea for a research or training project will be competitive for funding. Funding agencies have specific areas that they want studied. You also have interests that you want to pursue. It is when these interests intersect that funding may occur. Therefore, you may have to modify your research idea to match the interests of a particular funding agency. Alternately, you might find, after an extensive search, that no agency is funding topics in the area you have identified. If this is the case, you need to find a new area of investigation.

A third point to consider is the systematic nature of grantsmanship. The purpose of grantsmanship is to build a program of research or training. Each grant proposal you write should be a stepping stone for the next one you plan to write. In other words, a grant proposal should be one component of a planned program of research or education. A mistake frequently made by novice investigators is that they find an interesting project and try to obtain funding, but then shift their work effort to a different area of interest. This approach will result in a series of disjointed projects that may not produce more than small amounts of money and, more importantly, will not fully contribute to knowledge building.

A fourth point is that grantsmanship should be considered an integral part of your professional responsibilities. This is particularly true for faculty members in a university setting. Research, teaching, and service are all fundamental components of your career. The same is true, although to a lesser degree, for those in practice settings, where external funding can improve opportunities to advance practice or offer innovative services. Whenever possible, you should make grantsmanship complementary to other job responsibilities, rather than view it as a separate and distinct effort. For example, if you are a faculty member, you might think of what you can learn from your teaching and service activities that suggest an area of investigation. The courses you teach will immerse you in the research literature that may suggest an important topic for a research study.

Developing a research career is usually accomplished in a series of interrelated steps, each building on the one before. Ask yourself, "Where do I want to be 3, 5, or 10 years from now with respect to my research career?" This may initially be a difficult question to answer. However, developing proficiency at research and gaining funding for your ideas takes time and patience and involves a focused effort and well-defined goals.

Let's look at a fairly common situation and see how one faculty member might approach finding funding for a project that interests her.

1.1 A GRANT STORY

Ms. L. is an assistant professor of social work at an urban university. The school in which she works has departments of physical therapy, occupational therapy, and nursing. Ms. L. volunteers in a number of homeless shelters throughout the city and has organized a student volunteer program. In her volunteer work, she notices that shelter residents have significant health problems and difficulties accessing social services. She is convinced that a formal educational program to prepare social work, nursing, and allied health students to work in these shelters is essential to help alleviate some of these problems. Unfortunately, she doesn't know how to go about developing such a program.

Ms. L. decides to meet with her department chairman to inquire about recruiting more students to work in the shelters and to suggest that the department offer a formal educational program. At the meeting, her chairman points out that, while Ms. L.'s idea is a good one, starting a new program is expensive and time consuming. Since the school is short of both money and faculty, the chairman tells her that it is not possible to invest the department's limited resources into a program such as this. The only way that such a program could be supported would be for Ms. L. to find money elsewhere to pay for its development and implementation.

During her next evening of volunteer work, Ms. L. becomes even more determined to do something about the health problems she sees. The next day she makes an appointment to meet with a senior faculty member, Dr. A., who has received grant funding for a number of projects. She explains her idea and asks for advice. Dr. A. is sympathetic, but tells her that because of her inexperience she will have to be patient and develop a systematic plan to pursue funding for this project. He suggests conducting a literature review to learn the magnitude of the health problems that exist among shelter residents locally and nationally, the major problems that residents have accessing social services, and whether or not other programs in operation address this problem. He also recommends that she write up some of her findings and make them known to the professional community. Finally, he suggests that she "cast a wide net" in her search for a funding agency since her inexperience will make it difficult to obtain funding from the larger, well-known federal agencies such as the National Institutes of Health (NIH). He also suggests that she work with others who are more experienced grant writers. These people would not only help her gain experience, but their participation on her grant team would strengthen grant applications and enhance their competitiveness.

Ms. L. then meets individually with senior faculty members in the departments of nursing, occupational therapy, and physical therapy. She explains the problems she has seen in the homeless shelters and asks if they would be interested in helping her write a grant proposal to obtain funding for an educational program to prepare students to work in the shelters. All of the faculty members express great enthusiasm and suggest that Ms. L. call a meeting once she has identified potential funding sources. Ms. L. agrees and sets out to do her homework.

Where does Ms. L. begin her search for funding? Her first step would be to learn the basic language of grantsmanship.

1.2 THE LANGUAGE OF GRANTSMANSHIP

As in other fields, there is a specific language that is common to grantsmanship. It is important to learn this language in order to understand the grant writing process, communicate with agency personnel, and interpret application instructions for submitting a proposal idea. Here are 14 terms that are commonly used in the funding environment and throughout this book. These terms, listed in Box 1-1 and defined below, will help you get started in understanding agency language and communicating with those in this environment.

BOX 1-1

14 COMMON TERMS IN GRANTSMANSHIP

a. Research grants
b. Training/educational grants
c. Demonstration grants
d. Agency
e. Call for proposals
f. Competition
g. Preferences, priorities/special considerations
h. General instructions/supplemental instructions
i. Grantee/grantor
j. Principal investigator/project director
k. Program officer/project officer
l. Peer review panel
m. Pink sheets
n. Funding cycle

a. *Research grants*—Research grants provide money for an investigator to conduct a specific scientific inquiry, either basic or applied. In basic research, an investigator examines a question that will add to the theoretical body of knowledge in a discipline. In applied research, the investigator applies a specific theoretical principle, program, or approach to a practical situation. A research grant will usually provide money for salary support of the investigator and his or her team; materials needed to carry out the research, such as laboratory specimens, chemicals, supplies, or mailings; data analysis; and travel to professional meetings. The grant may also provide stipends for graduate or undergraduate students. In some instances, the grant will also pay for the purchase of special equipment needed to carry out the project.

b. *Training or educational grants*—Training or educational grants are those which have, as a main purpose, the education or training of students, faculty, clinicians, or other practitioners. These grants are used for planning and implementing new undergraduate or graduate programs, revising or updating curriculum materials, recruiting students into special programs, or helping health and human service professionals gain new knowledge or develop new skills. They also provide money for salary, supplies, travel, consultants, graduate students and, in some instances, equipment.

c. *Demonstration grants*—Demonstration grants provide support to projects that evaluate a model program, set of services, or methodology. A demonstration project usually builds on existing knowledge that suggests a given model or service is an effective way to address a specific issue. These types of grants are most commonly pursued by health and human service providers who wish to expand existing services or develop innovative model programs that can be replicated.

d. *Agency*—The term "agency" will be used throughout this book to refer to any funding source. The reason for using the more generic term is that most funding sources have a variety of departments that are called by different names. For example, the federal government is divided into a bewildering array of organizational units called centers, offices, institutes, bureaus, divisions, departments, or administrations, all of which may have programs of funding. Private foundations have different organizational structures through which money is awarded. Private companies also have their own way of naming departments that provide support for projects.

e. *Call for proposals*—A call for proposals is a notice of an opportunity to submit a proposal on a specific topic. Agencies publish announcements describing a problem area and inviting interested parties to propose ways to investigate all or part of the problem. These announcements vary considerably in the detail of their descriptions of projects they would like to see submitted. The federal government tends to provide very explicit descriptions of what needs to be included in grant proposals. Foundations and private companies tend to be much more general.

f. *Competition*—The term "competition" will be used throughout this book. It simply refers to a particular grant program for which a call for proposals has been issued.

g. *Preferences, priorities, and special considerations*— Frequently, a federal agency will decide to fund proposals that give special attention to a specific issue related to the area they want addressed in the call for proposals. For example, some agencies are interested in funding projects that are interdisciplinary in nature or that focus on underserved populations. When this is the case, the instructions will indicate "extra credit" will be given to proposals that include a focus on these approaches. There are three categories for which extra credit may be given, *funding preferences, funding priorities,* and *special considerations.*

In competitions with a *funding preference,* special attention is given to applications that address the stated preference. For example, if preference is given to problems in underserved communities and your proposal meets this requirement and is approved for funding, you will be funded before other approved applicants who do not meet the preference. If you qualify for a *funding priority*, the score assigned to your proposal will usually be adjusted favorably by a predetermined amount, such as 5 or 10 points. In competitions that include a *special consideration*, reviewers have additional latitude in assigning points to your proposal score. Each agency decides whether or not to use one or more of these funding mechanisms, although in some instances one is required by the authorizing legislation for that particular grant program. If one or more of these mechanisms is offered, you should seriously consider trying to qualify. Although not required for approval, it will make your application more competitive. Be sure to state in your proposal that you are requesting a preference, priority, or special consideration and describe the specific reasons why.

   h. *General instructions/supplemental instructions*—General instructions provide guidelines for submitting a grant application. These guidelines must be followed very carefully. Most general instructions address the following types of information: the date the application is due; the address where it should be sent; the required number of copies; the content of each section of the application; an identification of any preferences, priorities, or special considerations; the amount of money available; and the average expected funding range of projects. The general instructions might also include the guidelines used by reviewers who will evaluate your proposal and the number of points given to each section. Supplemental instructions extend or modify the general instructions for a grant application. These also must be read carefully because the agency may have made significant changes in the requirements for a proposal after the general instructions have been printed. Your application may be less competitive if the supplemental instructions are not followed.

   i. *Grantee/grantor*—The grantee is the institution or individual who submits the grant application and receives a grant award. A grantor is the agency providing the grant funds.

   j. *Principal investigator/project director*—The principal investigator is the person who will direct a grant project. This title is used most often in research grants. A project director is the term applied to the person directing a training, educational, or demonstration grant. In both cases, this is the person who oversees the grant activity, assures the scientific integrity of the endeavor, and is responsible for assuring that the grant is conducted in accordance with all conditions and regulations.

k. *Program officer/project officer*—A program officer is an employee of a federal agency who manages a specific program of grant funding. A project officer is someone who is assigned to supervise and provide technical assistance to a particular funded grant.

l. *Peer review panel*—A peer review panel is a group of experts selected by an agency to evaluate grant proposals submitted in response to a call for proposals. The panel evaluates each proposal and makes recommendations to the agency as to which should be funded. Each agency may use and structure panels in different ways. The structure and composition of panels within the federal government are determined by statute or other federal guidelines. The National Institutes of Health, for example, select individuals who represent different knowledge areas, such as health services, behavioral science, or medical research. These panels are called initial review groups (IRGs) or study sections. Members are appointed for specified periods of time (usually three years) and usually meet three times a year to review proposals. Other agencies may select panels for one particular competition. All of these panels may vary in size from three to perhaps 15 experts. A number of different formats are used when convening review panels. This is discussed further in chapter 11.

Many private foundations do not use peer review panels. Decisions regarding funding are made by the board of directors or the trustees of the foundation. Their decision is often based on the evaluations and recommendations made by program officers who work for the foundation. Proposals may also be reviewed by foundation work groups or committees of experts who are convened for a specific competition.

m. *Pink sheets*—"Pink sheets" are written evaluations of proposals that are sent to principal investigators or program directors. They are named, quite simply, for the color of the paper on which they were once printed. The pink sheet usually provides an in-depth narrative assessment of your proposal, including an overall summary of the strengths and weaknesses, the panel's critique of each section, and recommendations or suggestions for improvement. Careful attention to this critique is important because, if you are not funded, the critique can provide some insight as to whether or not your application is likely to be funded if you revise and resubmit it at another time.

n. *Funding cycle*—Most federal competitions are on a funding cycle. This cycle refers to the due dates of applications for a funded program. Many federal agencies have funding cycles that occur at the same time each year. For example, in the NIH system, there are three deadlines for submitting individual investigator research grant applications (commonly referred to as an RO-1: October 1, February 1, and June 1. Information on submission dates can be found on the web site of an agency.

1.3 DEVELOPING A PROFESSIONAL GROWTH PLAN USING A RESEARCH CAREER TRAJECTORY

Now that you have an idea of the basic principles of grantsmanship and know key terminology, it is important to consider ways to prepare yourself for a research career involving grantsmanship. Developing your research career should be part of a long-range plan for professional growth and development. Writing a grant proposal represents a significant investment of time and energy. It should, therefore, be an activity that enhances your career and professional goals. It is important to remember that developing skill in writing a grant proposal is compatible with the goals of a health and human service professional.

As we discussed earlier in this chapter, when you identify an idea for a grant proposal, you should also think about what you want to accomplish in 2, 3, or 5 years. A grant proposal, especially if it is funded, should be part of a larger plan that provides incremental personal and professional growth and experience. Box 1-2 outlines four components of a strategy for professional growth.

BOX 1-2

COMPONENTS OF A PROFESSIONAL GROWTH STRATEGY

1. Build individual credentials
2. Build a track record of funding
3. Work on teams with more experienced researchers
4. Develop a plan for long-range, personal development

Let's look at each of these strategies individually.

1. *Build individual credentials*—Building your credentials requires time and patience. When you submit a grant proposal, the peer review panel will look closely at your credentials as part of the evaluation process. For example, Box 1-3 contains a typical comment by a review panel regarding the credentials of an investigator who did not demonstrate sufficient expertise in the topic of his proposal: congestive heart failure and a nursing home care intervention.

BOX 1-3

The principal investigator, Dr. T., has a Ph.D. in sociology and is an assistant professor. His past experience has included extensive research in gerontology and health care interventions for stroke patients. However, he has no previous research experience or publications on nursing, home care, or congestive heart failure. There is no doctorally prepared nurse on the project, which is also a problem. In particular, the team lacks clinical research expertise with congestive heart failure patients. The project would be enhanced by collaboration with nurses who have both clinical and research expertise in this area.

Building your credentials in a field can be accomplished in the following ways: 1) presenting papers at professional meetings; 2) developing these presentations for publication; 3) writing a book review or column for your professional newsletter; 4) serving as a reviewer of abstracts for a professional meeting; and 5) serving as a reviewer for a grant competition.

2. *Build a track record of funding*—Part of building your personal credentials involves developing a funding track record. Once you have identified an idea and a funding agency, you also need to show the agency that you are capable of successfully implementing the idea. Funding agencies require that an applicant demonstrate that he or she has the expertise to carry out the proposed project. Therefore, they will look for what is called a "track record" or prior successful experience in the content area for which funds

are requested. This track record is usually evaluated by the number of professional presentations and publications you have in the area, or by previous funding experience.

3. *Work on teams with more experienced researchers*— Another important strategy to enhance your credentials and improve your grant writing skills is working with others who have more experience than you. If you find an investigator who is planning to submit a proposal, volunteer your services. Offer to assist the team in ways that fit with your skills and make a contribution. You will find that most experienced investigators will welcome your help if you have something to offer. Becoming a member of an investigative team will also give you a track record in grant work and allow you to obtain important insight regarding how proposals are written. If the proposal is funded, you will also gain invaluable experience in the administration of a funded program. Take the time to learn from these more knowledgeable investigators.

4. *Develop a plan for long-range, personal development*—To develop a plan for professional growth, begin with an outline of your career or professional goals. Ask yourself the following questions: 1) What do I want to be doing three to five years from now? 2) Am I more interested in research, teaching, or clinical work? While research, teaching, and clinical work are interrelated, you may want to place more emphasis on one of these areas. The area you select will then influence the type of grant you choose to develop.

As you identify your career goals and develop your plan, talk to your supervisor, department head, and/or director. Engage in a dialogue that clarifies their expectations and goals for you, and for the department and the institution as a whole. From these discussions, you will have a better idea of how compatible your goals are with those of your department or institution and you will get a sense of the amount of institutional support you are likely to receive as you pursue grant funding. These discussions will also help you decide on the types of grants to explore. For example, if you are interested in curriculum development and your department values and supports educational innovation, then you will probably receive the institutional support necessary to pursue a training grant. If, on the other hand, your department has a greater interest in research, you will need to rethink your goals and perhaps develop your research skills or examine your curriculum interests from a research perspective.

The following is a description of an approach to developing a research career growth plan that encompasses these points.

A RESEARCH CAREER TRAJECTORY

Successful grantsmanship involves a step-by-step progression; you build on your expertise and develop credentials as a research scientist or educational trainer as you move forward. It is a rational and systematic process. In Figure 1-1 we outline a systematic approach to developing a research career. This Research Career Trajectory is most appropriate for those in faculty positions. However, many of the activities are relevant for individuals in practice settings as well, particularly those involved with the professional activities described in the initial career building stage. Also, a similar trajectory can be followed for building a career as a funded educator/trainer.

As you can see from the Trajectory, building a research career is a planned series of highly interrelated and iterative steps that move you from novice, to intermediate, to advanced, to expert levels of research and grant writing skill. Each level is composed of three fundamental activities. These include the following: making presentations at professional meetings, publishing in professional journals, and conducting research. The number of activities you undertake, and the depth to which you engage in them, will change depending on your level of expertise along the Trajectory. There are a number of ways to accomplish each of these key activities. You may not need to use all of these.

The time frame for moving from novice to intermediate to expert will vary, depending on a number of factors. These include the match of your research idea with the interests of a funding agency, your success at gaining funding at various stages, and a certain amount of luck. This Research Trajectory is a guide for thinking about and planning your grant writing career in a systematic way. It is also a helpful tool for mentoring others and/or in department planning.

NOVICE

At the novice level, your primary goal is to identify a research area of interest that is broad enough so that it allows you to develop meaningful questions and build a strong program of research. This requires that you initially identify a broad area of inquiry within which to examine more specific research questions. Let's say you are interested in issues related to the functional capacity of individuals with dementia. Your first step is developing researchable questions that address one part of this broad area of investigation. For example, as a health professional, you find that it is difficult to evaluate physical function in persons with dementia. The accuracy of reports of daily functioning provided by either a caregiver or the person with dementia is unclear. The research literature suggests that caregivers tend to over- or underestimate functional capacity depending on their own level of stress. Thus, one researchable question would be, "What caregiver characteristics, other than stress, may have an impact on the accuracy of proxy reports?" Another question you may evaluate is the relationship between performance-based measures and self-report measures of physical function.

A similar process needs to occur if you are interested in developing an educational or training program for students or practitioners in a particular area. A broad educational idea may be identified, such as training health professionals in early intervention programs for children. A grant application might then focus on one aspect, such as testing the effectiveness of web-based strategies or interdisciplinary approaches to such training.

At the novice level you need to engage in other important activities. These are making presentations at professional meetings, publishing in journals, and seeking money for pilot studies. Let's examine each of these activities:

Presentations and Publications

As a novice, it is critical to start with a comprehensive literature review on your topic. This literature review will help you become familiar with the current state of knowledge in the field. You will learn what research has been conducted in your area and the gaps that exist in the knowledge base. It will show you the kinds of research questions that are being asked in the field as well as the research designs and measurement instruments that are most common.

A literature review is an on-going process that you must continually engage in at each step of the research trajectory. Once the literature review is complete, you will be able to determine the primary issues in your area of interest and some of the significant research questions suggested by the gaps in the knowledge base. This is one way to identify a broad area of inquiry and, within that, narrow your focus to a researchable question.

From the knowledge gained from your review, you may be in a position to develop an abstract suitable for presentation at a professional meeting. One approach may be to identify a gap in knowledge and make recommendations regarding how to address it. Another might be to apply a particular theoretical framework to a practical situation to explain why a specific technique works in practice. Another approach may be to present an innovative teaching technique that you have developed and found to be effective. At this point in your career, you should target your local professional association and submit abstracts for presentation at their next meeting.

The next step would be to use this presentation as a base, expand on it, and turn it into a short article that you can submit for publication. Again, at this stage in your career, the most appropriate places to submit your manuscript would be smaller, local or state journals or even professional newsletters.

Another strategy would be to contact one of the journals or publishers in your field and offer to review books for them. Publishers are often eager to receive reviews of new books reviewed by those in practice or teaching. Some journals also have special sections that introduce readers to the latest works in a particular area of inquiry. Publishers, and some journals, provide you with a copy of the book to review.

Some journals also publish summaries/abstracts of recent relevant published articles to enable their membership to become aware of the latest thinking in the field. Conducting these reviews can provide you with up-to-date information and, at the same time, give you a publication related to your research area of interest.

Research Funding

As a novice, you will also need to develop your skill in conducting research. One way to gain experience is to identify a funded researcher in your department or college and volunteer to work on his or her grant. Some investigators welcome the involvement of novice faculty in their research. You may be asked to conduct a literature review or engage in other related research activities such as interviewing subjects. This involvement will provide you with information about the day-to-day activities of a funded project, as well as experience working on a research team.

Another way to develop hands-on research experience is to seek out funding for a small research project. Based on your background reading, you should be able to formulate a question that can be studied on a small scale. Many universities have small pots of money earmarked for faculty development. This money might be available from your department chair or from your college. Usually, these are small amounts of money ranging from $500 to a few thousand dollars. Use these in-house monies to conduct a small pilot study that will provide you with preliminary data from which you can develop a larger study.

Each of the above strategies will provide you with special skills, a knowledge base to pursue your idea, and experience in conducting research. They will also provide you with some beginning qualifications in your research area that will help you become more competitive for funding as you move to the next phase of your career.

INTERMEDIATE

Now that you have established your basic research direction, it is time to think about refining it. Your next steps are to enhance your research question and engage in studies of relatively larger scope.

Presentations and Publications

As you advance in your career, you need to continue to give presentations at professional meetings and develop these presentations into publishable manuscripts. At this point you should target national meetings for your presentations and peer reviewed journals for your publications.

Another valuable experience at this stage of a research career is to serve as a peer reviewer for your professional journal. Most editors of professional journals need to identify individuals with expertise in specific areas to review manuscripts. Serving as a peer reviewer will give you exposure to the latest thinking in your field and a better understanding of the components of publishable manuscripts. In addition, critically reviewing manuscripts helps to hone your writing skills and avoid common mistakes in scientific writing.

Research Funding

If you have received seed money to conduct a pilot study, the results of this study can be used to identify a larger research study and justify it empirically. Most grant applications include a section in which the applicants must outline their previous efforts in the proposed area and empirical evidence to support the research question.

There are numerous opportunities for small pockets of money. Some of these are with your professional organization, whereas others are with the federal government. Many professional organizations offer small grant programs for which you might qualify. These awards tend to range from $5,000 to $50,000 for studies or projects of interest to the profession. Descriptions and requirements for these competitions are usually advertised in the professional journal or found on the association's web site.

At the federal level, many of the institutes in the National Institutes of Health have small award programs that are designed to help new investigators gain research experience. One of these is called the K01 mentored research scientists award. This award provides funds to support an experienced scientist in your area of research to act as your mentor. There are other opportunities as well. These include RO3 awards for small research studies worth about $50,000 per year or up to $100,000 for two years, depending on the Institute; and R-21 awards for exploratory planning or developmental projects. These programs are described on the web site of each of the Institutes.

The pilot data collected in your earlier in-house study will be important for these small grant or mentorship awards. Pilot data will make your proposal more competitive since reviewers like to see that you have already begun to investigate an area. These small grants are designed to prepare you to conduct RO1 grants, which are the main mechanism for funding investigator initiated research studies at NIH. These RO1 grants are awarded to experienced investigators who have a well-developed research program and preliminary evidence to support a larger study.

NIH is not the only source of funding. At this stage, you should also consider other funding sources. The U.S. Department of Education has numerous research, training and educational funding opportunities. For example, The National Institute on Disability and Rehabilitation Research in the Department of Education has a field-initiated program. This competition invites applications on topics identified by investigators as long as they are related to the overall goals of the agency. The Bureau of Health Professions in the Health Resources and Services Administration of the Department of Health and Human Services has many training and educational grant programs appropriate for health and human services professionals. Gaining experience in research and collecting pilot data are important activities at the novice and intermediate levels, and will prepare you for these competitions.

At this point in your career trajectory, you may want to target 2–3 agencies whose funding interests are similar to your area(s) of expertise; learn about their funding priorities and proposal requirements, and contact the project officers and other investigators who they are funding. There are at least three ways to develop a better understanding of an agency's goals. The first is to contact a Project Officer in an agency. We discuss ways to do this in more detail in chapter 2.

A second strategy is to attend a technical assistance workshop sponsored by an agency. Many agencies at the federal level conduct what are called "Technical Assistance Workshops" prior to the date when grant proposals for specific competitions are due. These 1- or 2-day workshops are free, but some are by invitation only. You can obtain information about these workshops either from the agency's web page or by asking a project officer. If the agency is conducting an invitational workshop, you must submit a letter indicating your research goals and specific research questions. This letter serves as an application. If there is a match between your level of experience, research goals, and the agency's areas of interest, you will be invited to attend. At the workshop, members of the agency staff will discuss the upcoming competition, provide information on the kinds of studies or projects that they are interested in, and talk about the major components of proposals. There is often time set aside for you to meet with project officers to discuss your ideas.

Professional organizations, such as the National Council of University Research Administrators, also hold technical assistance workshops. Similar workshops are also provided by professional associations at their annual meetings. Although some have a registration fee, these workshops provide opportunities for you to listen to presentations given by representatives from a number of federal agencies, who discuss the kinds of projects they are interested in funding, elements of a competitive application, and upcoming grant initiatives.

Another excellent way to learn about submitting proposals for funding is to serve on the peer review panel of an agency. Although NIH has standing panels in which experts who are funded by the agency serve for a three-year term, other agencies appoint panels for a single competition. Many of these agencies are required by legislation to construct review panels with geographic and ethnic representation, so they are often seeking peer reviewers. Contact an agency that interests you and inquire about the possibility of serving on one of these panels. They will send you an application form that will ask you to identify your areas of expertise or to write a brief letter outlining your experiences. Your application will be kept on file and when a competition is held in your area of expertise, you may be asked to serve. The experience you obtain from serving as a reviewer will help prepare you to write competitive grants. You will be able to see the range of proposal ideas that are submitted and common pitfalls to avoid. You will also have opportunities to meet other experts in your area, who may be able to help you as you advance your ideas.

ADVANCED

The advanced level is characterized by a well-developed research program. The previous grants that you have been awarded and the articles you have published, will suggest next steps for your research.

Presentations and Publications

Presentations at national meetings, publishing in journals, and networking with colleagues who have similar interests all remain critical activities. At this stage, however, these activities are more focused and systematically build on your previous work. It is also helpful to target international meetings for your presentations and develop key collaborations with colleagues in other countries.

It is at this point that you may receive invitations to present your research at national or even international conferences. In addition, you may be invited to present suggestions to other new investigators at the technical assistance seminars conducted by various agencies. Finally, many agencies periodically conduct long-range planning meetings to set future funding goals. These agencies will often invite many of their funded investigators to participate in these meetings. Involvement in these planning sessions will not only provide you with more knowledge about the agency and their priorities, but will also allow you to influence their future funding decisions.

Research

If you have not already done so, you should be competing for the larger grants, such as the RO1's and program grants in NIH, or the similar grant programs in other agencies that we discussed in a previous section.

If you have already received several RO1 grants from an institute in the NIH, or major grants from other agencies, you may be invited to serve on one of their standing peer review sections or ad-hoc review panels. The standing peer review sections represent a three-year commitment, during which you will review grant proposals in your field three times a year. These are prestigious appointments and provide you with continued networking opportunities as well as in-depth knowledge of how to write a competitive application and what the agency is interested in funding.

Large foundations, such as Robert Woods Johnson or Kellogg may also have research funding opportunities in your area. Since these foundations usually fund experienced investigators, you may want to consider their initiatives at this point.

EXPERT

The expert level is characterized by having an active research program underway with one or more active grants at any one time. Collaborations with other experts, nationally or internationally, participation in expert panels, keynote addresses, program projects, and/or multi-site studies are core activities at this stage.

Presentations and Publications

Your presentation and publication efforts should continue, since the results of your research should be very influential in your field and pave the way for even larger grant projects. You will also be invited to present your research as keynote speeches at various national or international meetings.

Research

Now, you might also consider applying for P50 grants, which are large, multi-million dollar center grants. In these programs you would have a number of grants under your supervision as well as a team of other researchers.

SUMMARY

In this chapter you have learned about the essence of grantsmanship, its language, and about the importance of building a career in research by developing a professional growth plan. Six important points were discussed:

1. The essence of grantsmanship is to seek money that is available from a variety of funding agencies and write a grant proposal to convince an agency of the importance of your project and your ability to carry it out.

2. It is important to know how funding agencies operate and the areas they are interested in funding.

3. There is a specific language used by those who write grants and it is important to learn this language to better communicate with individuals in funding agencies and colleagues in your field.

4. Grantsmanship is a systematic process. There are well-defined and discrete steps in pursuing external funding. Each grant proposal you write should be a stepping stone for the next one you write.

5. Grantsmanship is an integral part of your professional career, whether you are in an academic or practice setting. Gaining financial support from outside agencies can improve your ability to advance the body of knowledge in your field, advance practice, or offer innovative services.

6. Developing a research career takes time and patience, but can be accomplished in a systematic way through a series of well-defined and interrelated steps, each building on the one before.

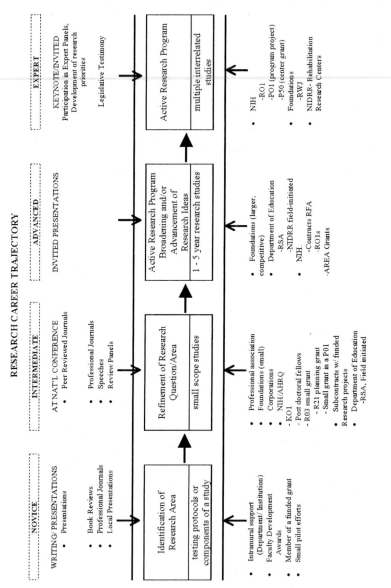

FIGURE 1-1

RESEARCH CAREER TRAJECTORY

Chapter 2

Becoming Familiar With Funding Sources

- Sources of Funding for Health and Human Services Professions
- Learning About and Keeping Track of Funding Sources
- Pilot Research Programs
- Interpreting Calls for Proposals

Now that Ms. L. has become familiar with the language of grantsmanship, her next step is to learn about potential sources of funding for her idea. Although identifying a competitive and scientifically sound idea for a project is critical, even the "greatest" idea will not be funded if it does not match the interest and priorities of an agency. Also, it is important to remember that once a notice or call for proposals reaches a public source such as the *Federal Register*, you may have only six weeks to develop a proposal. This may not be sufficient time to develop a competitive project idea and write a detailed, thoughtful proposal. Therefore, it is important to develop a plan to learn about the focal areas and types of projects various agencies seek to support. Since the funding environment and the interests of agencies are constantly evolving or changing, it is also essential to monitor changes in agency policies. Developing a plan of action is particularly important if your idea is in a formative stage.

In this chapter we identify the major sources of funding for health and human services professionals, discuss ways to learn about the current and future interests of various funding agencies, and suggest how to interpret the agency's call for proposals. Also, we emphasize pilot research programs that are particularly important for individuals in the formative stage of their research. Based on this information, you will be in a position to develop a plan of action.

2.1 SOURCES OF FUNDING FOR HEALTH AND HUMAN SERVICES PROFESSIONS

There are four major sources of grant funding for health and human services projects: the federal government, private foundations, professional organizations, and private industry.

BOX 2-1

FOUR MAJOR SOURCES FOR GRANT SUPPORT

- Federal agencies
- Private foundations
- Professional organizations
- Private industry

These four sources, discussed below, offer opportunities for funding a range of projects, such as small pilot research, conferences, demonstration projects, or large-scale education or research programs. In searching for funding, it is wise to cast a wide net initially. There are pockets of money available, often from seemingly unlikely agencies. Here we briefly describe each of these four sources.

A. *Federal government*—The federal government is a huge enterprise that is comprised of an array of departments, agencies, institutes, bureaus, and centers. The complexity of this bureaucracy can make it difficult for inexperienced investigators to navigate their way through this federal maze. Further complicating the situation is the dynamic nature of the funding environment. The priorities and interests of the various agencies are always changing in response to advances in knowledge, societal trends, and congressional activity. The federal government is, however, still the largest source of research and training money. The National Institutes of Health alone had a budget of approximately 27.3 billion dollars for 2002.

As you search for funding among the federal agencies, you will find that some may have interests which are, in general, similar to yours. You may also be able to identify agencies that initially appear unlikely to fund your ideas, but that may prove important to pursue in the future. For example, it is not uncommon for legislators to direct money for education or social services programs that benefit their constituents to federal agencies not usually associated with human services. These "pork barrel" projects are very common. For example, the *Washington Post* reported on March 28, 1995, that a $243 billion defense appropriation contained numerous non-defense programs, such as a $10 million national guard program to help Los Angeles youth and another $1.5 million to round up wild horses wandering on to the White Sands Missile Range. Agencies may also receive money for programs of particular interest or value to their employees. Again, the Department of Defense, which provides a variety of training programs for its employees, has received millions of dollars for studies on breast cancer. Similarly, the Department of Agriculture has had money in the past to fund many projects that one might expect to find in the Department of Education.

While there may be pockets of money for health and human service professionals throughout the federal government, there are two departments in particular that contain agencies with a focused interest in health and human service areas. These are the Public Health Service within the Department of Health and Human Services and the U.S. Department of Education. Within the Department of Education, the Office of Special Education and Rehabilitation Services (OSERS) has a variety of programs of potential interest to the health professions, as does the National Institute on Disability and Rehabilitation Research (NIDRR). The Fund for the Improvement of Post-Secondary Education (FIPSE), which is a foundation within the Department of Education, has many competitions that require innovative and generalizable approaches to educational problems.

B. *Private foundations*—Private foundations are also an excellent source of funding for health and human services projects. There are over 70,000 foundations in the United States that offer grants to individuals, institutions, or other non-profit groups. These foundations hold assets of over $150 billion and award over $8 billion a year in grants.

Foundations can be categorized into four types: independent foundations, company-sponsored foundations, operating foundations, and community foundations. Generally, only the first two types provide grants to independent investigators, although all four offer potential funding opportunities.

BOX 2-2

FOUR TYPES OF FOUNDATIONS

- Independent
- Company-sponsored
- Operating
- Community

---

1. *Independent* foundations have as their primary function the awarding of grants. The assets of most of these foundations are derived from gifts of individuals or families. Some operate under the direction of family members, whereas others are under the direction of a board of trustees. A Board of Trustees usually ensures that funds are spent for grant programs that were intended by the family. Still other foundations function more independently in awarding grants. The Pew Charitable Trusts and the Rockefeller Foundation are examples of two of the largest independent foundations. There are hundreds of other smaller foundations with interests in

funding projects relevant to health and human service providers.

2. *Company-sponsored* foundations have derived their funds from a profit-making company or corporation. They generally, but not always, award grants that are related to the business interest of the parent corporation. Two examples of these foundations are the Ford and Kellogg Foundations.

3. *Operating* foundations support research, social welfare, or other programs determined by their governing body. These foundations rarely award grants to outside organizations.

4. *Community* foundations derive funds from many donors. These foundations are often classified as public charities and generally limit their giving to charitable organizations in the local community.

C. *Professional organizations*—Your professional association is another appropriate source for obtaining funding. It is particularly useful for beginning investigators, since the interest of an association is to support the professional development of its members and conduct projects to advance the profession. Many associations provide small grants which may range from $2,000 to $50,000 or more.

D. *Private industry*—Drug companies, equipment manufacturers, and other companies related to health care often have money available for small projects. Many large corporations have funds for research projects that advance the interests of the company. The main interest of companies in the private sector is the testing or evaluation of their own products. For example, an oral health care company may need a new product tested for the prevention of plaque; an equipment manufacturer may need a new assistive device evaluated; or a company may pay for the development of a patient education video that promotes its product. The private sector is an untapped potential source of funding.

2.2. LEARNING ABOUT AND KEEPING TRACK OF FUNDING SOURCES

In searching for funding, it is initially best to "cast a wide net," and search for sources of support in both obvious and unlikely places. Where can you learn about funding opportunities? Here we describe *21* common sources used by investigators to learn about funding interests in the public and private sectors. These sources include those that are specific to the federal level, those that pertain to foundations and corporations, and those that are related to professional associations. If you are unsure of which agencies support your areas of interest, develop a search strategy that includes as many of these sources as possible.

    A. Federal Government

        1. *Program officers*—Perhaps the most valuable sources of information about funding are program officers who work in federal agencies. These individuals can provide invaluable assistance at all stages of the grant development process. Program officers usually have extensive experience overseeing grant competitions, know the type of project that will be most competitive in their agency, and are able to give you valuable suggestions about how to shape your idea to fit the requirements of a particular competition. In some cases, a program officer may be responsible for the development of the call for proposals and, therefore, will be able to provide specific advice about the type of project that the agency would like to see funded. Before you make a commitment to pursue a particular project, *call a program officer*. The name and telephone number of a program officer can be found in calls for proposals, in the *Federal Register*, or the *NIH Guide*. Often, the suggestions and advice these sources provide can result in the submission of a stronger proposal.

            Beginning investigators are often hesitant to contact a government official. However, program officers welcome calls and visits. Table 2-1 contains suggestions about what to say to a program officer when calling by telephone.

TABLE 2-1   What to Say to a Program Officer by Telephone

1. Indicate who you are
2. Give the name of your institution
3. Briefly describe your general idea and indicate the strengths you would bring to bear on a project
4. Ask if the agency supports a program in the area
5. Request an application kit and funding deadline
6. Ask if the program officer is able to review an abstract, concept paper, or draft of a grant application prior to submission
7. Ask if you can review proposals that have been funded in a prior competition, if you decide to visit Washington
8. Ask for a list of funded investigators whom you can then contact to discuss their research and whether they would share their grant application

When you talk to a program officer, identify yourself, briefly explain your idea, and ask if his or her agency might be interested in funding a proposal based on this idea. Also ask whether you can e-mail or fax a one- to two-page description of your project. In many agencies, a program officer will review this abstract or concept paper and inform you whether it would be appropriate to submit a proposal. If your idea does not fit the goals of the specific program announcement or agency, the program officer will let you know this as well, and might be able to suggest a more appropriate funding source.

You can also visit program officers in Washington, D.C. Unless an agency is in the middle of a peer review, you will usually be able to obtain an appointment. Table 2-2 presents seven suggestions to help you plan and conduct a visit with a program officer.

When you visit a program officer, plan for a 20–45 minute meeting. Before the meeting, learn about the kinds of projects the agency has funded in the past and their current areas of interest. The ways you can obtain this information are discussed later in this chapter. At the meeting, do not be reluctant to ask very basic questions, such as what the agency looks for in a grant proposal, how the peer review process works, what specific areas the agency seeks to fund,

TABLE 2-2   Visiting a Program Officer

A. *Before the visit*:

1. Review application materials and legislative priorities
2. Learn what kinds of projects the agency usually funds
3. Learn what projects the agency funded in the past two years

B. *What to ask during the visit*:

1. What are the common strengths and weaknesses of proposals submitted to the agency?
2. What are the major areas that will be emphasized by the agency in the current funding cycle?
3. What are the anticipated future areas of interest to the agency?
4. Can proposals that have been funded by the agency in the past be reviewed?
5. Can a grant application that is not funded be re-submitted?

---

and/or what competitions are upcoming. You will find that program officers are not only very helpful, patient and pleasant, but very candid about what you need to do to be successful. If you plan carefully, you may be able to visit three or four program officers in one day.

2. *Main information number of a federal agency*—Let's say you are unsure of which program officer in a particular agency would be most helpful for your idea. You can call the main number of an agency, and describe your idea in non-technical terms; the secretary will be able to direct your request to the most appropriate individual. Also, always check the web page of an agency to locate key information quickly.

3. *Catalog of Federal Domestic Assistance*—This is another important source of information about funding. This annual publication contains a listing of funding sources in the federal government. Each entry contains the title of a program, the name of the contact person, a brief summary of the kinds of projects that are funded, the amount of money that is available, the average size of awards, and anticipated information about the funding cycle during the upcoming year. To learn more about the catalog, go to the web page (http://www.cfda.gov)

4. *Monitoring legislation and government documents*— Monitoring the progress of major legislation is an important way of anticipating future funding initiatives. Congress appropriates money to all federal agencies with a general expectation that it will be used to investigate concerns of importance to the American people. For example, public concern regarding diseases such as AIDS and cancer have resulted in effective lobbying efforts on the part of special interest groups to support more research on these diseases. Congress has responded positively to this pressure and earmarked increasing amounts of money to address these problems. Since federal agencies must compete for funds, they often structure their planning agenda around issues of congressional importance. For example, some institutes in NIH have received increased levels of funding for basic research in cancer and AIDS. Other agencies that do not specialize in basic research may approach the problem of AIDS from a different perspective. For example, the Department of Education has an interest in funding AIDS education programs in the public schools.

One way to monitor legislation is to contact your senator or representative. When you visit Washington, D.C., make an appointment to discuss your interests and learn about the legislative agenda of your congressman. Appointments with a legislative aid are usually easy to obtain. These individuals will have detailed knowledge of the major issues on Capitol Hill.

You may also contact the government affairs office of your professional association. Members of this group will be monitoring legislation important to your profession and may be lobbying for a specific program of interest. They will also be very knowledgable about upcoming legislative issues.

5. *Congressional offices*—Your congressional representative can also help you locate appropriate funding sources. Write a letter to your senator or congressman, explain the nature of your idea, and ask for assistance in locating an appropriate government source of support. The health legislative aid of a congressman will

review your letter, label it "controlled correspondence" and forward it to one or more appropriate agencies. These agencies will then respond with suggestions. When writing this letter to your congressman, highlight how your proposed project may potentially benefit those in his or her congressional district.

6. *Federal Register*—The *Federal Register* is a daily (Monday through Friday) publication of the federal government. It provides a public announcement of regulations and legal notices issued by federal agencies. These include Presidential Proclamations, Executive Orders, federal agency documents that have general applicability and legal effect, documents required to be published by Acts of Congress, and other federal documents of public interest. Since all calls for proposals are listed in this publication, reading it will help you learn what agencies are funding programs in your area of interest. The office of the *Federal Register* often conducts workshops for the public that describe what the *Federal Register* is and how to use it. Information regarding these workshops is published periodically on page II. Online subscriptions are available to individuals for $300/year. To obtain copies of the Federal Register, write to: New Orders, Superintendent of Documents, P.O. Box 371954, Pittsburgh, PA 15250-7954. Call the order desk at 202-512-1800 or visit the website at http://www.gpo.gov/su-docs/aces/aces140.html. The cost for a copy is $8.00. Also, you can view the Federal Register at most libraries.

7. *Notices of upcoming competitions published for comments*—Prior to issuing a call for proposals for a major new competition, an announcement is printed in the *Federal Register* that invites anyone to comment about the scope and substance of the proposed competition. These announcements indicate that there will be an upcoming call for proposals in the area for which comments are sought. Anyone can respond in writing to the proposed priorities or suggest ways to improve the announcement. The agency evaluates each comment and responds to it in later editions of the *Federal*

Register. The final program announcement may be altered based on these comments. However, any changes will usually be minor and the final announcement will be similar to that which is finally published as a call for proposals. Therefore, reviewing these notices provides an opportunity for you to plan ahead and begin developing your proposal idea.

8. *Federal Grants and Contracts Weekly* and *Health Care Grants and Contracts Weekly*—For those of you who do not have access to the daily *Federal Register*, an alternative source is the *Federal Grants and Contracts Weekly* or the *Health Care Grants and Contracts Weekly*. These weekly newsletters summarize upcoming grant competitions that are appropriate for health care professionals. They also contain information about new federal or foundation programs. The cost is about $435/year for each. For a subscription, write to Capitol Publications, Inc., P.O. Box 1453, Alexandria, VA 22313-2053. The company also publishes newsletters devoted to funding opportunities in other disciplines, such as education.

9. *NIH Guide*—The *NIH Guide* is a weekly publication of the National Institutes of Health of the Public Health Service that announces upcoming grant and contract opportunities. It also provides policy and administrative information, such as requirements and changes in extramural programs that are administered by the NIH. While similar information is published in the *Federal Register*, the *NIH Guide* provides a more focused look at this group of funding agencies. The *Guide* is available electronically via the Internet (http://grants/nih.gov/grants/guide/).

10. *Commerce Business Daily*—The *Commerce Business Daily* (*CBD*) is a daily publication announcing federal grant and contract opportunities. Federal agencies, by law, must advertise contracts worth $25,000 or more in the *CBD* first. Referred to as the "federal government's official want ads," the *CBD's* primary mission is to publish requests for proposals. In the past, the *CBD* was predominantly used to solicit contracts. However, more recently, agencies are using it to

attract grant proposals as well. This publication is very comprehensive in that it publishes over half a million solicitations, worth over $200 billion, each year. Your library or office of research administration may have the most up-to-date copies of the *CBD*. Also, visit the website http.//www.fedbizopps.gov/.

Because the *CBD* is so comprehensive, it can be very difficult to review. A second option is to subscribe to a weekly summary, called the *Commerce Business Daily Weekly Release* (http.//www.fedbizopps/CBD weekly). This publication is a customized summary of solicitations published during the preceding week. You may select certain areas such as education, health care, or clinical research and receive a customized listing of solicitations in these areas. This summary is available from United Communications Group, 11300 Rockville Pike, Suite 1100, Rockville, MD 20852-3030. There is also an on-line order form.

Although contracts can be a source of funding for health professionals, the application process and the technical requirements are different than those of grants, and discussion of them is beyond the scope of this book. For information, contact Commerce Business Daily, Commerce Department, Washington, D.C. 20230, (202) 482-0732. For subscription information, contact the Superintendent of Documents, Washington, D.C. 20402-9238, (202) 783-3238.

11. *Serving on peer review panels*—Agencies frequently try to identify qualified professionals to serve on peer review panels. Serving as a peer reviewer is an invaluable experience in that it provides a great opportunity to learn about the characteristics of successful and unsuccessful grants and to enhance your skills at grantsmanship. The process of becoming a peer reviewer differs in each agency. In some agencies, particularly those within the Department of Education, you can submit your curriculum vitae with a letter requesting to be considered to serve on a peer review panel. In your letter, clearly identify your areas of expertise and the types of applications you believe you are qualified to review. The agencies will usually

send you a data form to complete, which they then keep on file. Being selected to serve as a peer reviewer is an honor and indicates that you are recognized as a leader or major contributor in your field. A program officer in any agency can inform you how to be considered to serve on a peer review panel.

12. *Serving on agency planning groups*—Agencies often convene planning meetings with their funded investigators. These meetings are designed to identify the current state of knowledge in a field and recommend new research or educational directions for the agency. Opportunities to serve on planning groups are usually reserved for individuals who have been previously funded by an agency. Once you are funded, inquire about such opportunities with your project officer. Often, an agency will publish proceedings from planning meetings and make these documents available. These can be very valuable sources of information since they provide a general long-range plan for the agency.

B. Foundations and Corporations

Foundations and corporations are another source of potential funding for health and human services professionals. With the anticipated and real cuts in federal spending, these funding sources are receiving increasing attention by those who formerly have been well supported by federal funds.

1. *Foundation Directory*—If you are interested in pursuing funding from private foundations, the best sources of information are *The Foundation Directory* and *The Foundation Directory, Part 2*. The Foundation Directory is considered the primary source of information on the largest grantmaking foundations in the U.S. It provides information on the 10,000 largest U.S. foundations. The Directory also includes over 46,000 grants to illustrate the interests of foundations. *The Foundation Directory, Part 2* details the next set of 10,000 large and mid-sized foundations and over 65,000 selected grants. Each entry in these directories include: the name and address of the foundation, a description of its general funding interests, a list of

officers and trustees, the types of grants and other forms of support that may be awarded, restrictions on programs by geographic location and subject area and application procedures. Although foundations do fund research projects, many are also interested in demonstration projects or projects that test a model program that can be replicated at other sites. Most university libraries have in their holdings the most up-to-date edition of *The Foundation Directory*.

Large foundations such as the Robert Wood Johnson Foundation or Kellogg Foundation often fund medical and health related projects. However, these foundations tend to fund experienced researchers or those that have received funding before. A good source for the inexperienced investigator are smaller foundations, which offer funds for pilot efforts or small projects in health care.

To help identify smaller foundations, use *The Foundation Directory, Part 2*. Both directories can be ordered from The Foundation Center, 79 Fifth Avenue, New York, NY, 10003-3076, and are available on CD-ROM.

2. *Foundation annual reports and newsletters*—An excellent supplement to *The Foundation Directory* is the annual report of a foundation. The annual report provides detailed information on projects which were supported during the past year. Past project funding is one of the best indications of the current interests of the foundation. Many also publish newsletters that describe ongoing projects and announce upcoming initiatives. To learn more about these opportunities, write or call a foundation and ask that your name be put on their mailing list.

3. *Annual reports of corporations*—If you are interested in pursuing funding from the private sector, an excellent source is the annual reports of corporations. Many large corporations, particularly the Fortune 500 companies, have offices of research that conduct studies of interest to the company. If your expertise or area of interest is related to that of the corporation, you might

be able to collaborate on one of these studies. In some instances, these offices pursue funding from outside sources. In other instances they are supported by the company. Annual reports provide information on the amount of money a corporation has devoted to research or educational projects during the last year. It also contains the names and telephone numbers of those to call for more information.

C. Professional Associations and Other General Sources

1. *Professional associations and newsletters*—The newsletters of almost all professional associations publish information on upcoming federal or foundation grant programs. They also provide information about their own grant programs. In addition, some associations have an office of research that helps locate potential funding sources. Others have a governmental affairs office with staff members that spend a significant amount of time on Capitol Hill and are knowledgeable about upcoming funding opportunities and current legislative initiatives. These offices are important resources for keeping abreast of changing funding trends.

2. *Professional meetings*—When you attend the annual meeting of your professional organization, talk to funded investigators. These individuals are usually willing to talk about their grantsmanship experiences and offer advice on potential funding sources. Associations frequently sponsor workshops on proposal writing at annual meetings that involve participation of representatives of federal agencies. Such forums provide valuable information about current trends and future directions.

3. *Agency advisory committees*—Many professional associations appoint members of the profession to committees that advise federal agencies. For example, an advisory committee composed of health professionals from a variety of disciplines was convened to help shape the priorities of the National Center for Medical Rehabilitation Research. If your profession is participating in these activities, they

may be tracking the funding priorities and can provide firsthand information about the future directions of many agencies.

4. *The professional literature*—As a faculty member or practicing health professional, you need to keep current in the professional literature. Knowing the trends in research or education in your profession and area of expertise will help you anticipate new funding directions. These trends often become reflected in the funding environment and, therefore, help you plan for future calls for proposals.

5. *Electronic databases*—Many funding agencies are developing or using electronic databases to disseminate information about new initiatives or calls for proposals. Private companies have also developed database programs that allow you to learn about funding sources. Some offer comprehensive services to help faculty members match an area of interest with a funding source. One example is a program called the Sponsored Program Information Network (SPIN). This is a database of funding opportunities designed to identify external support for research, education, and development projects. The database profiles over 5,000 federal, nonfederal, and corporate funding opportunities. It is designed to match an individual's research interests with funding opportunities through a key word index. SPIN is one of many databases that is available to aid in your search for funding. Your university library or office of research information can inform you of available databases.

6. *Newsletters in specialty areas*—There are other publications such as *Aging Research and Training News, Educational Bulletin,* or *The Chronicle of Higher Education* that routinely monitor funding opportunities in a focused area. A subscription to one or more of these sources is helpful.

2.3 INTERPRETING CALLS FOR PROPOSALS

Ms. L., in our grant story, has now used a number of these sources to identify potential funding opportunities. While scanning the *Federal Register*, she identifies a call for proposals in the area of her interest. But she is unsure how to interpret the instructions. She has also noticed differences between federal and foundation requests for proposals in the level of specificity of their directions. This is what Ms. L. needs to know in order to interpret a call for proposals:

Federal Government

To interpret a call for proposals, it is helpful to understand first how it is developed by an agency.

The first point to understand is that each federal agency is required to submit an operating budget to Congress that includes plans for the types of programmatic areas the agency hopes to initiate or continue to support. During the budget process, the President and each branch of Congress develop a budget that contains the amount of money that is recommended for authorization to each agency. After a period of budget negotiations, the final authorization is translated into an appropriation. The appropriation is either earmarked for specific programs or left to the discretion of the agency. The funds that are earmarked to a particular programmatic area are then used for the competitions that stimulate a call for proposals.

Generally, a call for proposals is developed by a program officer who spends considerable time and effort in conducting the necessary background work to support the area of inquiry. This background work may involve a thorough review of the literature, a review of findings from previously funded projects related to the topic of the proposed competition, commissioned or invited papers at conferences sponsored by the agency, major government reports such as *Healthy People 2010*, directives contained in major pieces of legislation, or long-range planning meetings sponsored by the agency.

Based on this information, the program officer develops a plan for a competition, which includes a justification of the importance and need for the topic and a description of how the topic fits with the mission of the agency and general interest of the Congress. The plan is then reviewed and revised by others in the agency until there is general approval. The revised plan is then published in the *Federal Register* and comments from professionals in the field are invited. Based on these comments, the agency decides if revisions are needed in their initial plan. At this juncture, an agency will know how much money they have to spend, the types of projects they are interested in funding, and approximately how much money can be targeted to each program area. From this information it is relatively easy to compute the number of projects they expect to fund. All of this information will be included in the final published call for proposals.

As a potential applicant, it is important to know that the call for proposals is well thought out and that a program officer has been closely involved in its development. Knowing this makes it incumbent upon any potential applicant to stay current in the literature of his or her field as well as knowledgeable about major government reports and legislation, since these will be the major sources used in the development of a competition. Because the Program Officer is usually closely involved in the process, he or she will have a very good idea about which project ideas may be the most competitive and match the intent of the call.

Once you obtain a call for proposals, how do you interpret it? A call for proposals contains a description of the objectives of the projects that the agency wants to fund, the types of organizations that are eligible to receive funding, detailed instructions on how to submit a proposal, and the due date of the application. The announcement may also contain information that will help you organize the presentation of your ideas, such as recommended sections for the narrative or the criteria used by reviewers to evaluate proposals.

If you are submitting a proposal to the Department of Education, the application forms will be found in the *Federal Register*. If you are submitting a research grant to the Public Health Service, you most likely will need to use the standard form, PHS 398. This standard application form can be obtained from the Division of Grants Management at the National Institutes of Health or, if you are at a university, from the office of research administration. Forms are also available electronically and in the near future most government agencies will require electronic submissions.

In fact, in the near future most grantsmanship activities will be conducted electronically. Many agencies have already adopted online submissions and do not accept paper copies of proposals. Some agencies are now requiring their continuation reports and other correspondence to be submitted online. In some instances, grant reviewers must obtain a grant application online and submit their review electronically. Although this will not affect the basic points discussed throughout this book, it will have implications for the way you compose and submit your proposal in the future. The changes brought about by advances in technology for the most part will make grantsmanship a little easier. However, it will require a different approach to planning and communicating with the funding agency and officials within your institution.

Benefits of Online Grantsmanship

Perhaps the chief benefit of the technological move towards online grantsmanship is the ease with which proposals and continuation reports can be submitted. Since an application can be submitted directly from your office, you will not have to be concerned about scheduling mail delivery, duplicating multiple copies, or rushing to the post-office or airport to deliver your application. This also translates into potential cost savings.

Another benefit is that you will have immediate access to application packages as soon as they are released by the funding agency rather than waiting for a mail delivery. Communication with program officers will be easier and more efficient. Instead of playing "phone tag," you will be able to leave email messages that can be answered at any time. Technology will continue to facilitate file sharing with colleagues at other national and international institutions much easier. This will be particularly important if you are involved in a multi-site study or cross-national project. The other main benefit of these technological advances is that there is greater access to the most up-to-date publications, government reports and news releases. Thus, it will be easier to check for the most timely information and statistics that are necessary to support a project. Additionally, with most journals moving to online access, writing a literature review for a grant will be much easier.

Potential Concerns

The transfer from paper to electronic grantsmanship does however present potential drawbacks or limitations. Since your institution will have rules about who needs to approve your proposal and provide the required signatures, adjustments will have to be made so the process is acceptable to funding agencies as well as your institution. Some agencies currently using online applications require that a letter from an official in the institution be faxed or mailed prior to accepting the electronic application. Other agencies accept the application, but require official documentation from the grantee's institution prior to making the award.

As with paper proposals, great care must still be given to writing and proof reading. Some people find it more difficult to work online and it may be easier to miss small mistakes. Remember that once you hit the send button, it is not possible to retrieve your proposal. Obviously, even with an electronic submission, you must allow sufficient time to submit your proposal. It might be wise to have a back-up plan in case your computer crashes, you are unable to access your application materials online, or your computer or network is not available. Also, you will need to make sure your computer has sufficient capacity to handle large files, since most applications and their instructions may be large. Finally, it is wise to contact your institution's technology services to assure that you have the correct software to read and overwrite on electronic applications. Find out what type of emergency services are offered by your technology to help create your back-up plan when writing and submitting the proposal.

In some cases, online submissions do not save money. You still need to print out all the files, proofread hard copies of the application and duplicate hard copies for inter-office records. Obtaining the correct application forms and downloading also can take some time and can be frustrating if you do not have the correct software.

Application Kit

Some announcements for competitions indicate that an application kit needs to be requested from the agency or downloaded from a website. This kit contains the application forms and a Program Guide that describes the rules and regulations of the competition and the information that needs to be included in each section of the proposal. These are very important documents, which must be read carefully before you begin to write your proposal. You must always follow the suggested outline provided by an agency and organize your application according to the evaluation criteria that are often provided in the application kit. Box 2-3 provides an example of information from an application kit for the Allied Health Projects Grant competition sponsored by the Bureau of Health Professions.

BOX 2-3

I. Background and Rationale

    A. What is the purpose of the project in relation to the legislative purpose (Section 767, PHS Act)?

    B. Is a background statement of the national/local need for the proposed project included?

    C. Is the proposed project an appropriate, innovative, effective, and efficient means of addressing the problem?

    D. Are the background statement and rationale appropriately researched and referenced in the proposed project?

II. Objectives

    A. What are the objectives?

    B. Are the objectives clearly and concisely stated?

    C. Are the objectives stated in measurable terms and achievable?

III. Project Methods

    A. Are the methods/activities clearly related to the objectives of the proposed project?

    B. Are the methods/activities to accomplish the objectives clearly stated? How will the activities be implemented and accomplished?

    C. Have necessary commitments from cooperating institutions been obtained? For example, letters of support and memoranda of agreement.

    D. Are the methods/activities outlined in the proposal the most effective to accomplish the objectives?

    E. Are the methods/activities clearly assigned to the responsible staff? Cooperating institutions?

    F. Is there a feasible timetable of the work plan included with the proposal?

Table 2-3 contains a list of the criteria that the Bureau of Health Professions has used to evaluate proposals submitted in response to grant programs.

TABLE 2-3

- The extent to which the proposed project meets the legislative purpose
- The background and rationale for the proposed project
- The extent to which the project contains clearly stated realistic and achievable objectives
- The extent to which the project contains a methodology which is integrated and compatible with project objectives, including collaborative arrangements and feasible work plans
- The evaluation plans and procedures for program and trainees, if involved
- The administrative and management capability of the applicant to carry out the proposed project, including institutional infrastructure and resources
- The extent to which the budget justification is complete, cost-effective, and includes cost-sharing when applicable
- Whether there is an institutional plan and commitment for self-sufficiency when federal support ends

---

If you submit a proposal to this agency, you need to become familiar with the legislative purposes of the competition and demonstrate that your proposal addresses its intent. The proposal should satisfy each of the elements of the evaluative criteria shown in Table 2-3.

Sometimes agencies publish supplemental instructions. These contain changes to program requirements that have been made after an initial Program Guide has been published. The supplemental instructions may either modify or supplement the requirements in the original set of instructions. The supplement may also contain a more detailed outline of the review criteria that will be used by the review panel so it is important to pay close attention to such changes.

In some instances, agencies provide advance notice of the competitions they expect to fund in the upcoming year. For example, the following information found in Table 2-4 was extracted from an announcement in the *Federal Register* (Vol. 66, No. 5,

January 8, 2001) submitted by the Department of Education, Office of Special Education and Rehabilitative Services, National Institute on Disability and Rehabilitation Research (NIDRR). This announcement invited applications for new disability and rehabilitation research projects for Fiscal Year 2001–2002. In the announcement, NIDRR described the required proposal sections for the two competitions and the point value that would be used in their evaluation. Program #1 refers to the National Center on Accessible Education-based Information. Program #2 refers to the Disability and Business Technical Assistance Centers.

TABLE 2-4   Program

		Program #1	Program #2
a.	Importance of Problem	7	7
b.	Significance	—	3
c.	Design of training activities	24	14
d.	Design of dissemination activities	24	21
e.	Design of technical assistance activities	22	21
f.	Quality of project services	—	10
g.	Quality of management plan	3	3
h.	Adequacy of budget	4	4
i.	Quality of project evaluation	3	3
j.	Project staff	13	14

This table demonstrates the point values assigned to each section among the programs. The distribution of points identifies those sections of most importance to the agency. To be competitive, your proposal would have to be particularly strong in the sections with the higher point values. This is not to say that you should ignore those sections with low point values. For example, to apply to either program #1 or #2, it would be important to expend considerable effort to ensure that your project had a detailed and effective plan for dissemination since this section is worth 24 and 21 points, respectively. If, on the other hand, you developed a proposal for program #1, you would also give special attention to describing the training activities (worth 24 points) in addition to its technical soundness (worth 22 points). In program #2, two of the sections, dissemination and technical assistance, have relatively high point values (21 each).

For some competitions, an agency may request a "letter of intent" to officially inform them of your intention to submit an application. A letter of intent contains a statement that you plan to submit an application and a brief description of the program idea. These letters provide the agency with an indication of how many proposals they may anticipate and allow better planning as to how to organize the peer review process. It also enables the program officer to provide feedback about your initial ideas. This letter does not commit you to submit a final application, nor will you be evaluated on this idea and told not to submit an application.

FOUNDATIONS/PROFESSIONAL ASSOCIATIONS AND CORPORATIONS

Each foundation has its own procedure for administering programs of funding. Foundations are less constrained by regulations regarding the types of projects they can fund, the way they must process grant applications, and how they make funding decisions. For many foundations, the instructions for submitting a proposal are much less detailed than those of the federal government. Usually a foundation asks for a two- to five-page letter describing the project concept. They will then consider this letter carefully and, if they are interested, invite you to submit a full proposal.

The lack of detailed instructions does not indicate that foundations have less rigorous expectations about the quality of a grant application than other agencies. The same care needs to be taken with proposals to a foundation as with federal grant applications. As with a federal agency, you need to convince the foundation that your project idea is important, that you are the most qualified person to carry it out, and that it fits with the interests of the agency. Prior to submitting a concept paper or letter, it is critical to talk to a program officer in a foundation about your idea.

Professional associations will vary in the detail and format of their application procedures. If you decide to apply to your association, ask for their application kit or guidelines and read and follow them carefully. The main office of your professional association may also be able to clarify the questions that you may have.

Obtaining corporate support is a different process than gaining federal support. There are more than 160,000 companies that have assets of over $500,000. Each is a highly complex organization with many budgets that could be tapped. Because of this complexity, it is beyond the scope of this book to do more than summarize some suggestions for working with corporations.

Schumacher (1994) cites four distinctions between corporations and federal agencies that make approaches to gaining funding different:

1. Federal granting agencies are required by law to spend a certain amount of money on academic research. Corporations do not, and are in the business of making money.

2. Federal agencies publicize their external grant program. Most corporations do not even have an external grant program.

3. Federal agencies award a grant to an investigator they have not met. Corporations usually do not fund academic investigators they do not personally know and trust.

4. Only a handful of federal agencies fund individual investigators, while there is a vast number of potential sponsors in the private sector.

Obtaining funding from a corporation requires more than a great idea, an excellent research design, a well written proposal, and an experienced investigator. While these are important for success, more important is an investigator's ability to form a mutually beneficial and trusting research partnership with a company. Schumacher claims that the term "Partnership" means just what it implies; a truly egalitarian relationship in which trust is established and communication is maintained. As with all approaches to grantsmanship, the development of a partnership takes time and should start small and build slowly.

SUMMARY

In this section, you have learned about 21 sources that will help you to monitor and keep track of the changing funding environment. You have also learned how to interpret a call for proposals. Five points are important to remember:

1. The funding environment is constantly changing and, therefore, it is best to develop a systematic plan to monitor these changes and predict future funding opportunities.

2. Cast a wide net initially and examine many different funding sources. As you develop an understanding of the range of funding opportunities that match your areas of interest and level of expertise, your search will become more focused.

3. You may always contact a program officer at an agency to learn about a funding opportunity and to determine if your idea matches the interests of the agency.

4. Do not hesitate to talk to colleagues at professional meetings regarding their funding sources. Also, as you read the professional literature, pay attention to the agencies that are cited as supporting the development of the material presented in the article.

5. Always read, reread, and reread the application kit and supplemental instructions prior to committing your ideas to writing. Use the suggested outline or evaluation criteria provided in the application kit to structure the organization of your proposal.

Part II

The Perspective of the Grantee

The first step in grantsmanship is to understand the language of the funding environment and the potential sources of funding. The second step is to identify an idea that has the potential for funding. In chapters 3 and 4, we describe the process of grantsmanship from the perspective of the grantee, you, and your institution. Chapter 3 describes ways to identify an idea of importance to you and match it to a funding opportunity. Chapter 4 describes the information you need to know about your own institution or agency in order to submit a proposal and administer it, should a grant be awarded.

Grantsmanship is viewed as an activity that fosters an individual's personal and professional growth, as well as that of his or her discipline, department, institution, or agency. The identification of an idea and the steps necessary to develop this idea into a competitive proposal is presented as part of a broader strategy for personal and professional growth.

Chapter 3

Developing Your Ideas for Funding

- Identifying Competitive Ideas
- Which Ideas are Hot and Which are Not
- Matching Ideas to Funding Priorities
- Professional Growth Strategies

One of the most difficult aspects of grantsmanship is identifying an idea that has the potential for funding. While you may have many ideas that are interesting, important, or exciting, they may not necessarily result in funding. A **great** idea is just one ingredient of a competitive proposal. A great idea must still be shaped to adequately reflect the priorities of a federal agency, private foundation, or other funding source. However, you should not pursue an idea strictly on the basis of its funding potential. Any idea you develop must also be commensurate with your professional interests, area(s) of expertise, and stage of professional growth (see chapter 1, Research Trajectory). Thus, one of your first tasks in grantsmanship is to develop an idea that fits with your long term career interests, as well as the interests of a funding source.

3.1 IDENTIFYING COMPETITIVE IDEAS

Most professionals, whether they are academic faculty or practitioners, are able to identify areas in which they have a personal and professional interest. However, an idea that has funding potential must reflect national needs, the interest of your profession, and be operationalized concisely and cost effectively. Therefore, matching this idea with the interests and priorities of funding agencies can be difficult.

Developing an idea with funding potential requires creative and flexible thinking. The following are seven important sources which might help you formulate a competitive idea that has the potential for funding:

- Clinical or professional experience
- Professional literature
- Interaction with colleagues and funded investigators
- Societal trends
- Legislative initiatives
- Public documents
- Agency goals and priorities

a. *Clinical or professional experience*—A principal source of ideas for projects is your own clinical or professional experience. The challenges that emerge in classroom teaching, the persistent issues that arise in working with clients in a clinical setting, or problems identified in staff conferences or faculty meetings often yield critical questions that are worthy of investigation. For example, in one case, members of a department of occupational therapy noticed that a persistent topic in faculty meetings was a gap in knowledge and skills between academic faculty and clinical practitioners which often resulted in misunderstandings and conflict between these two groups. In discussions with colleagues, they found that faculty in other programs also had identified faculty-practitioner differences as an issue when providing clinical experiences for students. The identification of this issue stimulated members of the department to seek funds to create a training program that would link faculty and clinicians in a way that would minimize these differences and at the same time strengthen their relationship and enhance the skills of both groups.

After reviewing calls for proposals in the *Federal Register* and talking to program officers, two federal agencies were identified that appeared to have an interest in improving the relationship between faculty and practitioners: the Bureau of Health Professions (BHPr) in the Department of

Health and Human Services and the Office of Special Education and Rehabilitative Services (OSERS) in the Department of Education. One of the six topic areas of interest to the Bureau of Health Professions, Allied Health Special Project Grants for fiscal year 1993, was a request to develop "innovative models to link allied health clinical practice, education and research," (*Federal Register*, Vol. 57, No. 186, Sept. 24, 1992, p. 44190). In response to this announcement, faculty in the department of occupational therapy submitted a proposal to develop an inter-disciplinary curriculum in geriatrics that involved faculty-clinician teams from four disciplines.

Program officers in the Office of Special Education and Rehabilitation Services of the Department of Education also expressed interest in faculty-practitioner cooperation. Another proposal was submitted by the department to develop model clinical sites in which faculty and clinicians would collaborate as a team in training students involved in early intervention activities with preschool children.

b. *Professional literature*—Carefully reading the literature published in your field is an excellent way to identify topics with funding potential. Many professional associations establish both short- and long-term research and education goals for the profession and publish these in their national journals. They also publish policy statements and pertinent articles on current issues. All of these can be used as guides to identify and develop relevant ideas. Regional and national newsletters such as *OT Week*, *OT Advance* and *PT Advance* are also important sources of information about the current issues in each profession.

For example, *OT Week* periodically publishes a list of research topics that are identified by the American Occupational Therapy Association (AOTA) as important areas for investigation by the profession. These areas have included studies of the effectiveness of practice, cost-effectiveness and reimbursement considerations, program administration, educational improvement, inter-professional relationships, and instrument development. Although these are very broad topics, they identify the general areas of importance to the profession. These broad topics provide a starting point from which to develop specific research questions and projects. One of these areas, practice effectiveness, has also been identified as a funding preference by the American Occupational Therapy Foundation, which is the research branch of the profession. In this particular case, the profession not only identified a pertinent issue but also provided grant money to pursue it.

c. *Interaction with colleagues and funded investigators—* Your daily interactions with colleagues might suggest problem areas or issues that could be developed into fundable projects, as the example of the occupational therapy department discussed above exemplified. Topics that consistently emerge in staff meetings and other discussions often warrant systematic evaluation through a research or education project. Involvement with individuals from other disciplines, particularly those who have been funded, is another important source of ideas. Often, these discussions uncover common educational and research issues that are experienced by more than one health profession. In addition to inspiring fundable ideas, professional interactions, especially those that lead to collaborative relationships with those in other disciplines, may result in programs and proposals that are interdisciplinary in nature. Many federal agencies and foundations encourage these collaborative, interdisciplinary approaches in their calls for proposals. Interactions with funded investigators can be another source of ideas. These individuals can provide insights as to how agencies and reviewers critique ideas in a given area. They may be able to offer suggestions as to the best way to present an idea to reviewers based on their prior funding and review experiences.

d. *Societal trends—*Societal trends or concerns are also important sources that can help identify a competitive grant idea. These trends often signal the possibility that Congress may allocate money to address problems that stimulate these concerns. Consider the national focus on the high cost of health care. The health care reform debate has stimulated many federal agencies to focus on the cost-effectiveness of health care programs, alternative financing mechanisms, and programs of managed care.

For example, when the spiraling cost of health care first emerged as a national issue, the Agency for Health Quality Research (AHQR; formerly the Agency for Health Care Policy and Research) invited applications for research on programs of managed and coordinated care, with an emphasis on costs, quality, and health insurance reform (*NIH Guide*, Jan 29, 1993). Many other invitations for research or demonstration programs to test the cost effectiveness of a range of health care programs and health care practices have since been announced and this area of concern will continue to dominate the focus of numerous grant competitions. Foundations are also influenced by these societal concerns. For example, the Robert Wood Johnson Foundation has a long-standing and ongoing interest in health service delivery models, particularly for chronic care and home health care. They began by providing funding for the development of a theoretical framework for chronic care management. Currently, their initiatives focus on testing components of the model.

e. *Legislative initiatives*—Since legislative initiatives fuel the funding priorities of federal, state, and local government agencies, it is important to track and examine proposed and pending legislation. For example, the landmark Americans with Disabilities Act (ADA) of 1990 granted critical civil rights to individuals with disabilities. A major component of the Act required certain federal agencies to provide technical assistance to help organizations understand the ramifications of the ADA. As a result, the Department of Education sponsored a competition that funded a network of 10 ADA technical assistance centers. The Department of Justice also awarded grants for projects aimed at implementing components of the Act (*OSERS*, Vol. V, 32, 1992). Although technical assistance is no longer the primary focus of funding in the Department of Education, other related issues concerning disability and societal integration are the primary focus of recent funding initiatives.

Another influential piece of legislation is the Rehabilitation Act of 1973 (PL 93-112) which, in its most recent version, is called the Individuals with Disabilities Education Act

(IDEA). Based on the IDEA, the Department of Education sponsors periodic competitions for research studies, in-service seminars, model education programs, and training activities. These competitions involve a range of health professions including occupational therapy, speech therapy, special education, and physical therapy. A related legislative act, the Technology Related Assistance for Individuals with Disabilities Act of 1988 and its subsequent amendments have also influenced the development of numerous funding competitions in the National Institute on Disability and Rehabilitation.

As you can see, if you have expertise in an area covered by the ADA, there would be a number of funding opportunities to explore. However, you would need to revise your thinking as the focus of grant programs shifts over time as a consequence of funded project results and hence, knowledge building. Also, you need to keep abreast of the amendments and re-enactment of the major legislation, since changes in the act influence funding priorities and spur new areas of investigation.

f.   *Public documents*—Public documents and reports by major governmental agencies may also signal impending initiatives. The subjects of the reports and their recommendations can provide major clues to future funding initiatives. One key document for health professionals is the Public Health Service report, *Healthy People 2010: National Health Promotion and Disease Prevention Objectives* (to obtain a copy of this document you can go to the following web site: http:www.health.gov.healthpeople). This document has influenced previous and current funding, and will influence future planned funding priorities of many government agencies. Federal agencies under the Public Health Service use this report as a guide, and usually request that proposals address one or more of its priorities. Most grant program announcements will refer to this document. Take for example a research program announcement entitled "Telehealth Interventions to Improve Clinical Nursing Care," sponsored by the National Institute of Nursing Research and the National Library of Medicine (PA number PA-00-138, September

22, 2000). As in similar program announcements, it includes the following statement:

"The Public Health Service (PHS) is committed to achieving the health promotion and disease prevention objectives of "Healthy People 2010," a PHS-led national activity for setting priority areas. This Program Announcement (PA), Telehealth Interventions to Improve Clinical Nursing Care, is related to one or more of the priority areas. . . ."

In the Bureau of Health Professions, Allied Health Project Grants, applicants are instructed to describe the relationship of the objectives of their project to the achievement of the objectives outlined in *Healthy People 2010*. This is a clear message that your proposal must address these identified national priorities if it is to be competitive.

Other documents to be aware of are those published by the Institute of Medicine. For example, one of their documents, *Allied Health Services: Avoiding Crises*, has served as an important source of project ideas for health and human service professionals since 1989. This report addresses such issues as: a) predicted personnel shortages, b) the need to attract professionals from underrepresented groups, c) making health careers more attractive, d) strengthening education programs, e) retaining health care workers, and f) avoiding regulations that impede entry into careers. Each one of these issues can still be the basis of a competitive proposal.

g. *Agency goals and priorities*—Most funding agencies, whether in the private or public sector, set yearly goals and priorities. Many develop long-range plans which specify the types of initiatives they believe are important areas for investigation. These may be published in a variety of ways. Therefore, it is important to contact the funding agency directly to inquire as to whether a document that describes their long-range plans is available for distribution. Also, the annual reports of foundations usually contain a list of priorities and funding activities. These are important sources from which to learn of funding interests and the types of projects that have received grant monies.

3.2 WHICH IDEAS ARE HOT AND WHICH ARE NOT

As you examine the seven sources described above, you will begin to see trends that will help identify ideas that are "hot," or of particular interest to funding agencies, and those that are not. Box 3-1 outlines some of the key areas for which funding is currently available and those ideas or issues that are no longer of equal significance for funders.

In keeping with changes in health care, recent funding priorities reflect an emphasis on testing new models of care: those that are community- and home-based, interdisciplinary, and those which examine health promotion and disease prevention strategies. Newly implemented federal regulations mandate the inclusion of women and a wide range of minority groups (e.g., Hispanics, Asians, Russians, African Americans) or others who traditionally have been underserved (e.g., rural elderly, urban poor elderly, homeless, American Indians, Pacific Islanders) by the health care system. Funding agencies are also encouraging applications from "teams" of professionals, or center grants that involve individuals from widely different disciplines (e.g., biologists, economists and sociologists). Other foci include research and training programs that address critical shortages in the health care workforce. Also of interest are programs that are capable of leveraging resources such that more than one source of funds is used to build or expand on a project, and programs that demonstrate self-sufficiency after funding is terminated. A relatively new focus of the PHS is research programs to identify factors that foster the rapid translation of research into practice settings. Funding to support the development and testing of translational research models is increasing. Finally, there is an increased interest by funders in applications that propose ideas that are portable and reproducible or which close the research-training-practice gap.

As you begin to identify your area or topic of interest, think of the current funding trends and how you can frame your idea accordingly.

BOX 3-1

WHAT IS HOT	WHAT IS NOT
• Community and home-based service models	• Hospital-based systems
• New health care models (cost-effective patient outcomes)	• Unidiscipline research, service, education approaches
• Underserved populations	• Narrow focus on minorities
• Innovative use of technology	• Exclusion of women
• Chronic disease self-management	• Research with little clinical applicability
• Workforce issues	• "Doc-top" models
• Informal caregiving	• Specialty training programs
• Translational research	• Large overheads
• Interdisciplinary team approaches to service, research, education	• Operating costs
• Innovative health promotion, disease prevention programs	• Programs needing continued support
• Leveraging funds	
• Self-sufficiency	

3.3 MATCHING IDEAS TO FUNDING PRIORITIES

Let's say you have used one or more of the seven sources we have described to identify an idea for a proposal. You have also conducted a search and found the agencies that are most interested in your identified area. What is your next step? Matching your idea with a funding interest takes time and creative thinking. It means framing your idea in such a way that it not only reflects contemporary thinking, but is also of interest to the agency you have selected. Here are seven steps you might follow to match your idea with the interest of a funding agency:

First, identify a broad topic area through literature searches, discussions with colleagues, and the other sources we have described above. Ask yourself these four questions:

1. Is this idea stimulating and important enough to me so that I would want to spend considerable time thinking and reading?

   *If your answer is **NO**—find another idea. Even if there is a funding source available, it is not worth pursuing the idea if it does not fit into your overall professional goals and growth strategy.*

2. Does the idea reflect contemporary thinking in the field?

   *If your answer is **NO**—then maybe the idea is interesting but really not that important or is one that has been addressed and answered in the literature. Consider reading more on the topic in order to more fully understand the state of knowledge and accurately assess the gaps in understanding.*

3. Does this idea have long-term potential to be expanded and contribute to my career path?

   If you are unsure how to answer this question, consult with a colleague or your supervisor or director. Also, read more on the topic to understand where your idea fits within the broader field of inquiry.

4. What are the goals of my department, institution, and profession, and how do their goals fit with my topic of interest?

   A response to this question necessitates careful and detailed discussions with representatives of your institution. Let's say your institution primarily supports and values basic science research (e.g., discovery of a cure), and your research and/or educational interests focus on the outcomes of a disease process or technology as a vehicle for patient education. You may encounter some difficulty in obtaining the institutional resources and support necessary to pursue your area of interest. It is important to understand what is valued and what will be supported within your department and institution. It is also important for you to be clear as to what you would like to pursue and how that can be supported by your department and institution.

Second, based on your responses to the above self-study questions, develop a preliminary list of potential funding agencies. To develop this list, use the *Federal Register*, Catalog of Domestic Assistance, discussions with program officers, the *Foundation Directory*, and/or electronic databases or web sites.

Third, evaluate your resources by asking yourself these questions:

1. What is my level of expertise, interest, and comfort with this topic area?

   Refer to the Research Trajectory (chapter 1) to help identify where you fit along your career path and funding potential. Then determine what skills will be needed to carry out your project idea and conduct a self-assessment of your level of expertise. You will then know what areas of expertise you will need to include on a grant application to successfully carry out your program and whether you will need to hire consultants or develop a diverse project team. Also, you may need to seek pilot funding if you do not have a track record in the area.

2. Are others available to serve as collaborators to complement my level of expertise?

   If your idea is significant to those in your institution, then it should not be difficult to identify others with either complementary expertise or interest.

Fourth, in light of your responses to steps 2 and 3, begin to specify and narrow your area of interest.

Fifth, write an abstract or concept paper that reflects your current thinking. This will help you narrow your topic and force you to systematically describe your idea. This abstract or concept paper can also be used to obtain feedback from colleagues or program officers in a funding agency.

Sixth, contact the program officers from the list of competitions that you have identified. Discuss your ideas and determine if the idea fits the priorities of their agency.

Seventh, begin to reshape your ideas based on these conversations and a further review of the literature.

TABLE 3-1   Steps to Match Your Idea With A Funding Agency

STEPS

1. Identify broad topic areas
2. Develop preliminary list of potential funding agencies
3. Evaluate your resources
4. Narrow your area of interest
5. Write an abstract or brief concept paper
6. Contact program officers
7. Reshape your ideas based on conversations and literature reviews

The following scenario describes how this process might be carried out.

BOX 3-2

THE CASE OF MS. S.

Ms. S., who has a master's degree in occupational therapy, is a half-time faculty member. She has an interest in writing a proposal to obtain money to support herself for an additional 50% effort. During the previous year, she secured a $6,000 grant to develop a computer-assistive instructional package in anatomy for occupational therapy students. She also has had experience as a computer consultant on a funded educational program for vocational counselors working with patients with traumatic brain injury (TBI). Ms. S. wants to combine her interests and write a proposal to develop computer-assistive training materials for formal and informal caregivers of patients with TBI. What type of grant should she write and for what agency?

First, Ms. S. has two broad topic areas that interest her: the development of computer-assisted instructional programs; and helping formal and informal caregivers of those with traumatic brain injury. She conducts a database search for potential funding sources in these two areas, and simultaneously begins to assess her level of expertise. She also begins to think about ways to refine these interests.

As a result of her search and assessment process, she makes two discoveries. First, there appears to be greater interest from both federal agencies and foundations in community-based care models for individuals with TBI than computer-assisted instructional development. That is, most agencies appear more interested in testing model programs than in the development of computer-assisted training materials. Second, she realizes that she does not have sufficient expertise in project development nor substantive background in the area of TBI to submit a research proposal to the agencies that she has identified.

Ms. S. knows that if she wants to pursue funding in traumatic brain injury, she will need to increase her expertise. She decides that her best strategy will be to collaborate with someone with more experience and knowledge. She decides to approach Dr. J., who is the principal investigator of the funded project that involved Ms. S. as the consultant. Ms. S. suggests that her best role on a research study would be as a project manager, and offers to take the lead in developing the ideas and the grant application. Ms. S. also wants to examine the potential of using her expert knowledge in computer-assistive technology in this research project. Dr. J. is very receptive to this idea since it has the potential to extend her current grant and is compatible with her personal research goals.

Ms. S. and Dr. J. meet and discuss several possible ideas. Ms. S. reviews relevant literature and then writes a one-page abstract that she shares with other colleagues to obtain feedback. She then telephones the program officers of the federal agencies and foundations she had identified earlier. Based on these discussions, she refines her idea for a project and begins to develop her proposal in more detail.

SUMMARY

In this section, you have learned about sources for competitive ideas and how to match these ideas to the interests of funding agencies. Four key points were discussed:

1. There are seven major sources from which to identify an idea with funding potential and you should consider as many of these as possible in developing a research or educational project.

2. Even the best idea will not be funded unless it matches the interest of a funding agency. Competitive ideas must reflect both contemporary thought in a field and the interests of an agency.

3. It is important to stay abreast of current legislation in your field of interest and identify the areas that are "hot" or fundable and those that are not.

4. There are seven basic steps to help you match your idea with those of funding agencies.

Chapter 4

Learning About Your Institution

- Questions to Ask of Your Institution
- Institutional Review Board Procedures

As we discussed in chapter 2, funding agencies have detailed instructions, requiring careful attention, that guide the submission of proposals. However, your agency or institution also has rules about submitting a proposal that must be followed carefully. These rules concern how to obtain institutional approvals for submission of your grant application, what can be requested in a budget, and the requirements to obtain approval of your procedures for the protection of human subjects, if that is relevant for your project.

Your institution also has policies that need to be followed should your project be funded. These policies involve procedures about recruiting and hiring personnel, reporting grant-related expenses and submitting required reports. (We discuss these requirements in detail in chapter 13.) Therefore, knowing the policies and procedures of your institution early in the proposal development process will help you work productively at both the pre-award and post-award stages.

4.1 QUESTIONS TO ASK OF YOUR INSTITUTION

Here are the most important questions to ask your supervisor, department head or other administrators in order to learn about the rules of your institution or agency:

TABLE 4-1   Eight Questions to Learn About Your Institution

1. What are the procedures you need to follow to obtain approval from an official in the institution to submit a grant application? That is, who in your institution is officially permitted to sign the face sheet of an application? How much lead-time does that person need in order to approve your grant submission? What materials does that person require (internal forms, sections of the grant application) to review for approval?
2. Who in the institution needs to review and approve your budget? What resources are available to help you prepare a budget? How much lead-time do these individuals need to work with you and approve your budget? What is your institution's facilities and administrative rate?
3. If your application requires hiring new personnel, what are the procedures you will need to follow?
4. What is the required official information that is necessary to complete the application, including your institution's assurance forms, and the face page information such as congressional district number and contact information for the responsible institutional officials?
5. Once a grant is received, how are the funds administered? Which office monitors the budget and prepares the final budget reports that are required by the funding agency?
6. What are the institution's procedures for processing payment of grant expenses?
7. What are the policies regarding the distribution of Facilities and Administrative costs (F & A)?
8. What other policies exist that are related to the implementation of grants?

Let's examine each of these questions.

1. *What are the procedures you need to follow to obtain approval from an official in the institution for a grant application?*

   Although a grant, particularly for research, is awarded to the principal investigator, it is the institution that must assume legal responsibility for the conduct of the project and the expenditure of funds. Therefore, an official who is the legal representative of the institution must sign off on every application prior to its submission to an agency. Thus, you need to determine who in your institution must sign the face sheet of the application. Many universities have an "Office of Research Administration" that reviews all applications prior to their submission. Other institutions require that a draft of the grant be provided to the signing official a week or more in advance of its due date. Still others may require a meeting to discuss the grant prior to obtaining the official signature.

2. *Who in the institution needs to review and approve your budget? What resources are available to help you prepare a budget?*

   Developing a budget can be complex, especially if you are hiring consultants or entering into agreements with other institutions. In some institutions, an office of research administration or a budget administrator will provide technical assistance or actually develop the budget for you. Even if someone else in your institution assumes responsibility for creating your budget, you should learn the following information:

   • Fringe benefit rate of your institution

   • Allowable percent increase for yearly salaries of the funding agency and your institution

   • Salary figures for personnel on the grant

   • Facility and administrative (F & A) rate, also referred to as indirect cost recovery rate of your institution

   We discuss budget preparation and these issues in more detail in chapter 6.

3. *If your application requires hiring new personnel, what are the procedures you will need to follow?*

Although you may not need to know this information prior to submitting an application, it is still preferable to learn about your institution's personnel policies. The human resource or personnel department usually has stringent rules and regulations that need to be followed in hiring new personnel. This department can also show you how to write a job description that fits your requirements, how to advertise for the position, if necessary, and the salary range that would be appropriate and approved by the institution.

4. *What is the required official information that is necessary to complete the application, including your institution's assurance forms, and the face page information such as congressional district number and contact information for the responsible institutional officials?*

Most applications require that an official at your institution sign various forms, assuring that your institution meets all certification requirements, such as Civil rights compliance, Drug-free and Smoke-free workplace, and information about Lobbying, debarment and suspension. Consult with your office of research to obtain signatures for these forms. The face page or your application to federal agencies requires that certain information be provided. This information includes the number of your Congressional District, the identification number of your institution, and the contact information for the responsible officials at your institution. Sometimes all the formal required information for a grant application is posted on the web page of the office of research administration or updated yearly and circulated via memos to key administrators throughout the institution.

5. *Once a grant is received, how are the funds administered? Which office monitors the budget and prepares the final budget reports that are required by the funding agency?*

When you receive a grant award, your institution will usually maintain the official budget, disburse your funds, make the appropriate financial reports, and monitor your expenditures. However, you still need to maintain a working budget, so you should inquire about the kind of reporting you may be required to provide and how best to interact with the offices that provide oversight. For example, some institutions keep track of all expenditures and provide the investigator with periodic reports. Other institutions expect the department and/or individual investigator to establish an accounting mechanism, although all payments still have to be approved by the financial officer. The procedures that are followed in your institution will shape the way you manage your budget.

6. *What are the institution's procedures for processing payment of grant expenses?*

This information is important to know in order to meet your financial obligations, such as payment to other pay institutions and consultants, or for ordering equipment and other supplies in a timely manner. Each institution has its own forms, time lines, set of procedures, and requirements for official signatures. Knowing these procedures will help establish a structure in which to effectively administer your grant and expedite many of the administrative tasks.

7. *What are the policies regarding the distribution of facilities and administrative cost?*

In some institutions, the individual and/or the department that receives the grant is given a percentage of the Facilities and Administrative (F&A) costs to assist in administering the grant project. For example, let's say a department of physical therapy in a university receives a grant award for which the university will obtain a 60% F&A cost recovery rate. In some universities, 10 to 15% of the F&A costs are given back to the department to help off-set the additional, but hidden, costs associated with the administration of the award. In other instances, a percentage is given to the investigator to use as discretionary money. Investigators can use these funds to augment the direct costs associated with carrying out the project or may save these funds for future salary support of project personnel if there is a gap between funded projects. However, this policy differs among institutions and, in some settings, F&A costs are not shared with the investigator or department. These policies are important to know since they will affect how you think about and develop an appropriate budget, as well as how you develop a program of research over time.

8. *What other policies exist that are related to the implementation of grants?*

    As part of the planning for your first grant submission, set up a series of information-gathering meetings with key administrators or individuals in your institution that may have an involvement either in the pre-award or post-award phase of your grant. For example, the reference librarian will be an invaluable guide to information services that are available. Also, meet with your budget officer, key individuals in sponsored programs, the office of research administration, the office of the dean, and the department of human resources to discuss your grant program and how it might affect their departments. In addition to providing information about various administrative procedures that you must follow, these individuals might also be able to offer helpful suggestions that will save you time and effort if your proposal is funded.

4.2 INSTITUTIONAL REVIEW BOARD PROCEDURES

If you are developing a research proposal involving human subjects, you will need to submit your research protocol to your Institutional Review Board (IRB) for its approval either prior to the grant submission or within a designated time from the submission date or just prior to receiving the award, depending upon the agency and competition. In some institutions, the IRB is referred to as the Human Subjects Board or the Research Committee. According to federal regulation, an IRB or comparable committee must approve all government funded research involving human subjects. Most institutions extend this regulation to include any research, whether funded by an outside source or conducted independently of funding. Therefore, prior to conducting any type of research (pilot, non-funded or fully funded), IRB approval must be obtained. An IRB is composed of individuals with diverse areas of expertise in biomedical and behavioral research as well as consumers, who review each research protocol developed by members of the institution. The purpose of an IRB review is to ensure that the rights and welfare of study participants (and animals) in a study are protected and that the benefits of the research are greater than any risk associated with participation. The IRB evaluates each aspect of a research protocol including the consent form, advertisements for subject recruitment, data collection procedures, scripts describing the study to potential subjects, and the study design. The IRB also conducts an annual review of the progress of each approved research protocol to evaluate the number of subjects recruited, the incidence of adverse reactions, or the identification of new risks. Although you may view IRB procedures as stringent, this review is critical to assure proper research conduct and protect the rights of all human subjects.

Prior to submitting a research application, you need to learn about the procedures that have been established by your institution for IRB review and approval. If you plan to collaborate and recruit subjects from other clinical sites or universities, you will also need to discover what the institutional review board requirements of each of these sites are. While many clinical sites do not have a formal IRB, they will usually have some form of human subjects board, such as a committee that reviews and approves requests for conducting research on its premises.

It is also important to read the directions of a grant application carefully to determine when IRB approval is required (e.g., prior to the grant submission or just prior to the grant award). Some competitions require that IRB approval be obtained *prior* to the submission of the application although others stipulate that submission to, and approval by the IRB occur within 30 days of the grant submission. Still other competitions, particularly those sponsored by the Public Health Service, adopt what are referred to as "just-in-time" procedures. Under these procedures, investigators do not have to submit an IRB protocol to their institution until their application is recommended for funding. Even if IRB approval is not required prior to submitting your proposal, it is prudent to know what IRB forms must be completed. It is also wise to begin the approval process as early as possible because this process may take significant time.

Although each institution establishes its own set of procedures for the submission and review of research protocols, there are three different levels of an IRB review. The type of review—full, expedited, or exempt—you receive will depend upon the degree of risk associated with the research procedures. Each review will differ in the number and type of individuals who must read and approve the research protocol. A "full review" involves a review by all members of the IRB (perhaps 20 to 30 individuals). Usually, one member is assigned as the primary reviewer and one or more members are assigned as secondary and tertiary reviewers. The primary reviewer presents the protocol to the entire Board with input from the secondary and/or tertiary reviewers as to its strength and weakness. A full review is required if the research protocol involves one or more of the following groups or categories: a) infants/fetuses, b) children, c) pregnant women, d) prisoners, e) mentally incompetent individuals, f) addicted persons, g) HIV testing and AIDS, and h) research involving investigational drugs or medical devices.

A subcommittee that is appointed from the full board carries out an expedited review. Studies that qualify for an expedited review are those that involve only minimal risks to subjects. Examples of such research include: a) recording data from individuals 18 years or older using noninvasive procedures that are routinely used in clinical practice; b) using existing data, documents, and specimens; c) observation of individual or group behavior or characteristics of individuals where the investigator does not manipulate subjects' behavior and the research does not involve stress to the subject.

The chairperson or another appointed member of the IRB usually reviews research protocols that are determined by the IRB to be exempt. These studies are not monitored on a regular basis as long as the investigator continues to follow the protocol that was originally proposed, although informing the IRB of such research activity is mandatory. Categories of research that are considered exempt from full or expedited review include research involving the following activities: a) evaluation of normal educational practices, b) select telephone or face-to-face survey or interview procedures, c) observation of public behavior, or d) retrospective studies using secondary data sets or previously collected patient information.

Each institution establishes its own set of procedures for submitting research protocols to its IRB. Some require that an entire grant application be submitted to the IRB for review and that the principal investigator attend a meeting with the Board to present the study and respond to questions. Other IRB groups require that an abstract, informed consent, and responses to six basic questions be submitted for review. The basic information that most IRBs need in order to adequately review a study protocol is outlined in Box 4-1.

BOX 4-1

BASIC COMPONENTS OF AN IRB SUBMISSION
COVER SHEET:

Title of project, funding source, name of investigators, estimated budget and budget period, indication of use of human or animal subjects, FDA approved devices or drugs, signatures of key officials (investigators, department chairs, etc.), and assurance that the investigator has no conflict of interest in the study.

ABSTRACT:

Summary of the research, its significance and purpose, specific questions and hypotheses, recruitment procedures, subject inclusion criteria, and statistical analyses.

INFORMED CONSENT:

Consent form for use with all subjects in the study. A consent form outlines the study procedures in lay language, describes the risks and benefits to participation, and informs subjects of their right to withdraw from the study.

RESPONSE TO SIX QUESTIONS:

1. *What is the proposed involvement of human subjects and their characteristics?*
2. *What are the sources of research material obtained from individually identifiable living human subjects in the form of specimens, records, or data?*
3. *What are the plans for recruitment of subjects?*
4. *What are the potential risks—physical, psychological, social, legal, or other?*
5. *What are the procedures for protecting against or minimizing any potential risks?*
6. *Why are the risks to subjects reasonable in relation to the anticipated benefits to subjects?*

Let's examine the six questions in Box 4-1. These six questions must also be completed as part of the application process for all PHS grant submissions using the PHS 398 application form, as well and in human subject sections of grant applications for other agencies. These questions ask the investigator to specify the procedures of the study as they relate to the recruitment of human subjects, data collection, issues of confidentiality, and the risk/benefit ratio of study participation.

1. *What is the proposed involvement of human subjects and their characteristics?*

   This question asks the investigator to describe the study population and list and justify specific inclusion and exclusion criteria. If your study involves a special population, then you need to justify why this particular population is required. If your study excludes certain individuals, particularly women or minority populations, then you will need to justify their exclusion. Also, you will need to discuss the basic characteristics of the subjects you plan to recruit.

2. *What are the sources of research material obtained from individually identifiable living human subjects in the form of specimens, records, or data.*

   This question requires the investigator to identify the type of data that will be collected and the procedures that will be followed for obtaining information. Box 4-2 provides an example of a response to this question.

BOX 4-2

EXAMPLE DISCUSSION OF SOURCES OF RESEARCH MATERIAL

The primary source of research material involves two, two-hour personal interviews that will be conducted in the subject's home by a trained member of the research team at Time 1 (baseline) and Time 2 (4 months from baseline). The interview protocol will involve a series of structured and standardized scales reflecting domains such as functional level, depression, and health.

3. *What are the plans for recruitment of subjects?*

Here the investigator needs to specify the plan for recruiting subjects. If advertisements are used, then the IRB will need to approve the wording of all recruitment pieces to assure that they are not misleading or coercive in nature. Also, if compensation is provided to subjects, then a clear explanation of the procedures you will use, including how much and when subjects will be compensated is required. Box 4-3 provides an example of a response to this question.

BOX 4-3

EXAMPLE DESCRIPTION OF A RECRUITMENT PLAN FOR HUMAN SUBJECTS

Older adults living in the community will be recruited using a set of procedures that have been developed by the investigators and used successfully in other large-scale studies. These procedures involve the systematic outreach to an array of social services, medical centers, senior centers, and regional media sources using advertisements and letters inviting participation (see attached). Interested individuals will be instructed to contact the project manager by telephone. Eligibility will be determined by a brief (20-minute) telephone screen administered to individuals who call and express interest in study participation. This screen will determine level of functioning and difficulties experienced in carrying out daily activities, falls history, and mental status. For those individuals who are eligible to participate, an explanation of the purpose of the study, the time commitment, financial remuneration, randomization procedures, and nature of participation in the experimental and minimal treatment conditions will be given. A signed informed consent will be obtained in person by the research interviewer prior to the conduct of the first interview.

4. *What are the potential risks—physical, psychological, social, legal, or other?*

The investigator must indicate all potential known risks associated with participation in the study. In those studies for which there is significant risk, detailed information must be provided regarding the nature and extent of each risk and the statistical probability of its occurrence. Detailed documentation from the studies that have demonstrated these risks must be carefully described as well. Low-risk studies are much less problematic. Box 4-4 provides an example of a discussion of a low-risk study.

BOX 4-4

EXAMPLE DISCUSSION OF MINIMAL RISK

There is no known risk associated with participation in this study. There are no physical, psychological, social, or legal risks associated with the structured interviews. Occasionally, the content of the questions may raise personal and emotional issues for an older adult. Such responses to interview content, however, have not been found to pose a serious psychological threat. Interviewers are carefully trained to sensitively handle such issues and facilitate the participant's ability to successfully complete the interview.

---

5. *What are the procedures for protecting against or minimizing any potential risks?*

An investigator must not only identify all potential risks associated with study participation, but also develop a set of procedures to protect against or minimize the potential occurrence of each risk that is posed. As part of this discussion, the investigator should also describe procedures for maintaining subject confidentiality. An example is shown in Box 4-5.

BOX 4-5

EXAMPLE DISCUSSION OF PROTECTION OF CONFIDENTIALITY

Pre-coded data collection instruments will be prepared for use with subjects at each testing occasion. Identification numbers to assure subject confidentiality will be used. Only one master log containing the subject name, address, and telephone number and study identification assignment will be maintained. This log, in both hard copy and disk, will be stored in a locked filing cabinet separate from other identifying information. All completed data collection instruments will be stored in filing cabinets as well and kept locked in the researcher's office. Audiotaping of intervention sessions will be identified by numbers only and any transcriptions resulting from these tapes will not contain any references to names or other personal identifying information. Audiotapes will be destroyed at the conclusion of the study.

6. *Why are the risks to subjects reasonable in relation to the anticipated benefits to subjects?*

Finally, in this last question, the investigator is requested to explain why the anticipated benefits of the study outweigh the potential risks associated with participation. The investigator may explain the immediate benefits to subject participation (e.g., financial compensation, opportunity to participate in meaningful experience, opportunity to receive a new treatment), as well as the long-term expected outcomes (e.g., discovery of new drug or treatment that would benefit a clinical population or significant contribution to a body of knowledge regarding a disease).

Most studies involving human subjects will also require the use of an informed consent form. A consent form is a legal document that informs a subject about the study procedures and its risks and benefits. By signing this form, subjects acknowledge they understand that they have volunteered for participation and can refuse to participate or withdraw from the study at any time without penalty. Before you develop your own consent form, consult with your IRB to inquire whether there is a particular format or standard language that is required. Box 4-6 outlines the 13 basic elements that are included in any type of informed consent.

BOX 4-6

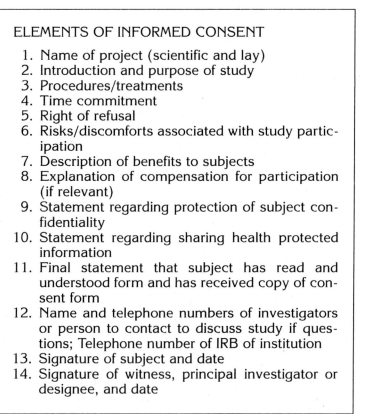

ELEMENTS OF INFORMED CONSENT

1. Name of project (scientific and lay)
2. Introduction and purpose of study
3. Procedures/treatments
4. Time commitment
5. Right of refusal
6. Risks/discomforts associated with study partic- ipation
7. Description of benefits to subjects
8. Explanation of compensation for participation (if relevant)
9. Statement regarding protection of subject con- fidentiality
10. Statement regarding sharing health protected information
11. Final statement that subject has read and understood form and has received copy of con- sent form
12. Name and telephone numbers of investigators or person to contact to discuss study if ques- tions; Telephone number of IRB of institution
13. Signature of subject and date
14. Signature of witness, principal investigator or designee, and date

1. *Name of project*—Informed consent forms often require two titles for a project, a formal title and then a lay title that can be understood by the public. Thus, investigators need to state the scientific title of the project first and then provide its translation into lay language.

2. *Study purpose*—The purpose of the study needs to be clearly stated, so that a lay person easily understands it.

3. *Procedures*—Each procedure must be accurately described so that a potential study participant understands the full extent of their participation.

4. *Time*—The time involved in each procedure as well as the length of time of the entire study needs to be described.

5. *Refusal*—Potential subjects must be informed that they have the right to refuse to participate in the study and that refusal will not effect their right to medical treatment or any other types of services. Also, subjects need to be informed of their right to withdraw from participation at any time without penalty, as well as their right to refuse to respond to interview questions.

6. *Risks/discomforts*—Potential subjects must be informed about any risks associated with participation as well as any discomforts that may be experienced. Each risk needs to be carefully explained along with a description of alternative treatments that may be available.

7. *Benefits*—An informed consent describes any immediate or long-term benefits to subjects. Benefits may include participation in a particular treatment, contribution to the research process, or other more tangible benefits that may be experienced.

8. *Explanation of compensation*—The compensation for study participation, if relevant, must be clearly specified so that a participant understands the circumstances under which they can expect remuneration.

9. *Subject confidentiality*—The investigator must discuss the procedures that will be used to assure confidentiality of the information that is collected. For example, the use of identification numbers to refer to subjects and keeping all subject data in locked filing cabinets are two important and traditional research procedures that should be discussed in a consent form.

10. *Health Insurance Portability and Accountability Act*—With the passage of the Health Insurance Portability and Accountability Act (HIPAA), it is now necessary to include

a statement in an informed consent as to how protected health information will be handled. You will need to indicate what specific information that is collected as part of your study will be shared and how it will be used.

SUMMARY

In this chapter, four major points have been made:

1. There are numerous regulations related to submitting a proposal and implementing a program that are specific to your institution. You need to identify early in the proposal development stage the procedures that need to be followed to obtain institutional approvals, the regulations associated with hiring of personnel and administering the budget, and other project implementation policies.

2. In addition to providing information about institutional requirements, administrators may also have helpful suggestions as to how to facilitate program development and implementation at the pre-award and post-award phases of your grant.

3. Protection of human subjects is essential in scientific research. Therefore, all organizations engaged in research have procedures to ensure that the participation of human subjects involves safe and ethical procedures. The Institutional Review Board is responsible for monitoring this aspect of research.

4. Each institution establishes guidelines for obtaining IRB approval. Information that must be provided includes the nature of the subject pool, the potential risks to these subjects, the benefits of participation, and the procedures that will be used to protect against or minimize these risks.

Part III

Writing the Proposal

The next four chapters contain the heart of the matter—writing the proposal. Each chapter covers a different aspect of writing, including an in-depth discussion of the basic sections of an application (chapter 5), a description of the elements of a budget (chapter 6), technical considerations and administrative matters (chapter 7), and strategies for writing effectively and concisely (chapter 8).

Writing and presenting your ideas in a concise, clear manner is one of the most important components of the process of grantsmanship. Proposal writing involves a style that is technical, crisp, and to the point. It is not an occasion to use a more literary, flowery, or embellished approach to writing. Unclear or confusing objectives, undeveloped methods, poorly referenced background and rationale, and vague evaluation criteria are all weaknesses that can be improved by attention to the process of writing a proposal.

Chapter 5

Common Sections of Proposals

- Description of Common Proposal Sections for Research, Training, and Demonstration Grants

Once you have identified a competitive idea for a research, education, or demonstration project, it is time to write the proposal. As with other aspects of grantsmanship, the writing of a competitive proposal is a systematic process. A proposal is simply a document in which you "propose" to carry out an idea. The proposal should present a compelling case to convince a funding agency to support your idea.

Agencies are interested in funding the best ideas from among those that are submitted. To help identify the best ideas, they provide you with the information that needs to be included in a proposal. This information, and the format in which it is presented, helps reviewers make judgments regarding the importance and quality of your idea and by which to compare one proposal to all the others that are submitted. Although each agency develops its own format for writing the proposal, there are sections that are common to most proposals.

5.1 DESCRIPTION OF COMMON PROPOSAL SECTIONS FOR RESEARCH, TRAINING, AND DEMONSTRATION GRANTS

The sections of a proposal can be thought of as a series of questions that you answer.

- What is your project about?
- Why is it important?
- What will you do?
- How will you do it?
- What will it cost?
- Why will it cost what it does?
- Why are you the best one to do it?

The instructions for a grant proposal can be thought of as a series of directions to help you answer these questions. If you keep these questions in mind and follow the directions of the agency as you write, it will help you focus on the important points you need to make for your application to be competitive.

As discussed in chapter 2, a federal agency informs applicants about the organization of a grant submission through its "call for proposals." Some agencies, particularly in the Public Health Service, publish a "Program Guide" that contains detailed information about what is expected in the proposal. Agencies will also occasionally issue "supplemental instructions" to this guide, if changes are made in their requirements after the program guide is in press or if a specific competition has additional requirements. You must always check to see if there are supplemental instructions. Supplemental instructions supersede and take priority over the instructions in the initial call for proposals. Other agencies, such as those in the Department of Education, publish an application in the *Federal Register* and include specific instructions for its completion. To submit to a foundation, you need to request an application kit. Most agencies, foundation and federal, now place their applications on their web pages. However, at this time, only a few accept electronic submissions.

The instructions for almost all competitions provide a comprehensive description of the proposal sections that are required, and usually specify the page length of each section and/or the maximum number of pages of the entire proposal. It is critical that the published guidelines from an agency be followed closely. In some competitions, you can lose points or, in the worst case, be disqualified from the competition, if you have not conformed to the agency's specifications. Therefore, prior to writing the proposal, read all the instructions very carefully to be sure that you understand the requirements. If you are unclear about the requirements of the grant submission, then contact a program officer to seek clarification.

A "call for proposals" or application kit often includes the rating system that will be used by the members of a review panel to evaluate your proposal. Some agencies may assign point values to each section of the proposal. As we discussed in chapter 2, the evaluative points indicate the relative importance of each section.

Although there is great variation among proposal formats, the sections that are commonly found in federal grant applications are listed in Box 5-1. Your responses to each of these sections should answer one or more of the questions we posed earlier:

BOX 5-1

- Title
- Abstract
- Introduction
- Goals/Objectives/Specific Aims
- Background/Significance/Importance
- Literature Review/Theoretical Foundation
- Methodology/Research or Educational Plan
- Dissemination Plan
- Plan of Management
- Investigate Team Credentials
- Institutional Qualifications
- Budget/Budget Justification
- References
- Appendix Material

Let's examine each of these sections.

a. *Title*—The title for your proposed project may initially appear to be simple to derive. However, it can be difficult to capture the main idea of your proposal in a short phrase. The title should describe the primary theme of your project so that it orients the reviewer to what he or she is about to read. It should not be so brief that it says nothing, nor so long that a reviewer has to work hard to figure out what it means. The following are examples of three titles.

BOX 5-2

Too brief:
"A Program to Help the Homeless"

Too long and convoluted:
"A Program to Understand the Health Care Needs of Those Who are Homeless by Working with Four Homeless Shelters and Developing Educational Materials for Students in Dental Hygiene, Nursing, Occupational Therapy, and Physical Therapy Programs"

Just right:
"A Community and Academic Partnership: A Program to Train Interdisciplinary Health Care Teams to Provide Services to Individuals Who are Homeless"

Many agencies now have specific requirements about the length of the title. For example, grants submitted to the National Institutes of Health (NIH), stipulate that the title not exceed 56 typewritten spaces, including punctuation and spaces between words.

b. *Abstract*—The abstract is a brief description of the proposal. Generally, the abstract contains a statement of the purpose of your study or project and a brief description of the research design or methods that will be used to carry it out. Agencies vary in their requirements. Many place a limit on the number of words that can be used (around 500). Therefore, the abstract must be very clear and succinct, but comprehensive. The abstract is very important, since it is the first section of the proposal that a reviewer reads and provides the framework for reviewing your proposal. An abstract that is not clearly written, that is not comprehensive, or that has typographical errors, can be misleading and give the reviewer a poor impression, potentially influencing how the entire proposal is evaluated. Because the abstract represents an executive summary of the entire project, it should be the last section you write. For NIH grant applications, the title and abstract are used by the

Center for Scientific Review to assign the proposal to a review panel. Thus, it is essential that both title and abstract reflect the core content of the proposal. The following is an example of an abstract.

BOX 5-3

EXAMPLE OF AN ABSTRACT

The purpose of this project is to develop, implement and evaluate a new program designed to educate physical therapy, occupational therapy, dental hygiene, and nursing students in interdisciplinary, community-based health care for homeless individuals. The program is based on a five-stage collaborative model which links allied health and nursing faculty, community organizations serving the homeless, and social workers in homeless shelters. The purpose of this partnership is to develop and implement innovative curricular activities for nursing and allied health students on interdisciplinary approaches to community health, including health promotion and restoration services. This three-year program will be carried out in three phases: a developmental phase in which a partnership will be formed among faculty and community participants; an implementation phase in which a curricular program in interdisciplinary community-based health care generated in the first phase is implemented; and an evaluation phase where the program is evaluated, the results disseminated to the academic and clinical communities, and the education model applied to other underserved populations.

c. *Introduction*—Most proposals begin with an introductory paragraph that provides the reader with a general overview of the main idea of the project and its importance. In this section you address what your project is about and why it is important. For example, the above abstract describes a proposal to develop a project that brings together university faculty and social workers to plan a curriculum to provide education for nursing and allied health students who are interested in working in homeless shelters. An opening introductory paragraph might discuss the increasing number of persons who are homeless in the United States and in the city in which the project will be held, the lack of health and social service personnel who are adequately prepared to work with this population, and the limited relevant curriculum content in the disciplines such as occupational therapy, physical therapy, nursing, and dental hygiene. Although this section is brief, it is necessary to cite data from sources such as national studies or reports and statements from professional groups.

d. *Goals/objectives/specific aims/activities*—If you are applying for training money, this section contains the goals and objectives of the educational program. There is often confusion as to the difference between a goal, an objective, and an activity. A training or educational program must be based on one or more goals. A *goal* is a statement that reflects what will be accomplished as a result of the program. It is a global or broad statement describing the overarching purpose(s) of the project or what you seek to achieve by conducting the proposed program. In turn, each goal has a specific set of objectives. An *objective* is a statement about a specific outcome of the program that can be evaluated or measured. Thus, it must be written in such a way as to reflect a qualitative or quantitative measurement strategy. For example, an objective usually includes words such as "increase," "describe," "reduce," or "enhance." Each objective is accomplished by conducting a number of *activities*. Thus, activities contribute to obtaining one's objectives which, in turn, lead to and define the goal. Therefore, if the activities are accomplished successfully, the objectives will be achieved, and the goal of the program will have been attained. An example of a goal, two of its objectives, and representative activities are shown in Box 5-4.

BOX 5-4

Goal: The goal of this project is to prepare future occupational therapists, nurses, physical therapists, and dental hygienists to collaborate in delivering health promotion and health restoration services in community shelters to persons who are homeless.

Objective #1: Increase the knowledge base of students in the biological, psychological, cultural, and social influences in providing adequate health services to persons who are homeless.

Activity: This objective will be accomplished through the following activities:

a. student participation in two specific departmental courses which provide the necessary professional knowledge, skills, and attitudes for working with the diverse population of individuals who are homeless.
b. student participation in three core multidisciplinary courses which relate theory, health policy, and research in the delivery of community-based health services.

Objective #2: Enable students to effectively collaborate as members of an interdisciplinary health care team.

Activity: This objective will be accomplished through student participation in two team-building courses, which are designed to move students from a uni-disciplinary to an interdisciplinary perspective.

If you propose to conduct a research study, then specific aims rather than objectives are presented. Aims are similar to objectives in that they stem from a research purpose statement and concisely describe what will be tested or evaluated in your research project. In addition to specifying the aims of the study, you may need to state hypotheses specific to each aim that you intend to formally test. These hypotheses, when tested, provide answers to the questions inherent in the aims of your study. An example of a specific aim and an accompanying hypothesis are shown in Box 5-5.

BOX 5-5

Specific aim: Test the immediate (3-months) and long-term (9 months) effects of a home-based skills training intervention for 250 caregivers of persons with dementia, using a randomized controlled two-group design.

Hypothesis: Caregivers of persons with dementia who participate in the home skill-building intervention will report reduced stress and burden in comparison to caregivers in a control group who receive education materials on dementia.

If you propose to conduct a study using a qualitative methodology in which formal hypothesis testing is not appropriate, then you will need to carefully explain this point to reviewers. Although there is increasing awareness among review panels of the scientific value of qualitative research, the formats for most proposals favor a quantitative or linear structure to describing the research plan.

If you are submitting an application to the National Institutes of Health, the specific aims section must not exceed one single-spaced typed page. This section should contain a brief statement of the research purpose, significance of the research problem, specific aims, hypotheses, and a brief statement describing the research design. It is imperative that you be very concise and clear in this one page since, along with the title and abstract, frames the entire proposal for reviewers.

For any application, the goal, objective, and/or aims statements are critical building blocks of a proposal. They provide the review panel with a mental template or a road map of what you plan to accomplish in the project. After you have written this section, ask yourself the questions presented in Box 5-6 as a way of reflecting on your work, and making sure that you have presented sound goals, objectives, or aims.

BOX 5-6

SELF-STUDY QUESTIONS

1. Are the goals, objectives and/or aims clearly defined?
2. Do the objectives, when taken together, define the goal of the study?
3. Are aims written as concise, testable statements?
4. Are key concepts/constructs defined?
5. Will the hypotheses, when tested, address the aims of the study?
6. Are the independent/dependent variables operationally defined?
7. Is the terminology used for the operational definitions clear and unambiguous?
8. Are the hypotheses/objectives stated in observable, measurable terms?
9. Are the hypotheses based on a sound theoretical framework?
10. Do the hypotheses clearly predict a relationship between variables?

e. *Rationale/significance/importance*—There is usually a section in a grant application in which you are asked to demonstrate the importance of the idea or its significance. Although having an idea that is exciting to you is a necessary starting point in writing the proposal, the idea must also be considered important to the funding agency. If a separate section on significance is not specified in the grant application kit, it is still in your best interest to find a way to inform the review panel of why your project is important. If a section on significance is not required, a strategic place to describe the importance of your project is in your introductory statements. After you introduce your idea, develop a logical, clear and compelling argument for why it is necessary. You need to make your argument persuasive, so that reviewers do not ask, "So what?". The "So what?" response represents a fatal flaw in a project. If a reviewer asks, "So what?" after reading your rationale, then your proposal has a poor chance of being funded, regardless of its scientific or methodological rigor.

In a training or education project, the significance of an idea is usually established by citing important research reports, professional literature, local and national data, and other government statistics that demonstrate a societal need for your project. If there is little data available, you may need to conduct a survey or needs assessment to document significance (see chapter 7). Even a small-scale or local survey helps to substantiate the need for and value of your program.

In a research project, the significance of the research idea is justified through a concise review of other research studies that highlight the level of knowledge in the field, the need for further research, and the ways your research addresses the gap in knowledge. Your review of previous research should demonstrate that your question is important, but one that has not been satisfactorily answered. Also, presenting preliminary findings from a small-scale or pilot study you have conducted on the topic strengthens the significance of your idea (see chapter 7). In the NIH investigator-initiated grant application using the PHS 398 form, there is a separate section for preliminary or pilot work.

You also need to state why and how your proposed study is innovative. Some applications will ask specifically for a section called "innovation." Although the PHS 398 application of the NIH does not specify a separate innovation section, the review panel is asked to comment on and evaluate the innovativeness of proposed studies. Thus, it is important to write a strong paragraph that explicitly states why your idea is significant and innovative.

f. *Literature review/theoretical foundation*—A review of the literature and description of the theoretical foundation of the study or educational program is often included as part of the significance section. In some applications, it is contained in a separate section. If you are writing a research proposal, it is important to show how the specific aim(s) and research question(s) are supported by a theoretical framework.

A theoretical framework should be clearly and explicitly linked to the variables you propose to analyze. A project that is based in theory will significantly advance the body of knowledge in that profession and strengthen your proposal.

In addition to a discussion of the theoretical framework, other relevant literature needs to be presented. The review of literature should be comprehensive and directly related to the topic of your proposal. It should include only the most pertinent and current works and not a long discourse about topics only peripherally related to your project.

There are five major reasons for reviewing the literature (DePoy & Gitlin, 1998). The first is to determine the extent to which your topic has been addressed in the published literature. If your research topic has been extensively investigated, you may need to reconsider either the importance of pursuing the topic or how you might modify it so that it systematically and logically builds on the existing empirical literature. If you are considering an educational or demonstration project and you learn that it has already been carried out, you will need to modify your ideas considerably. For example, you might develop a similar program but for a different population or setting.

A second reason for the literature review is to develop the rationale for the importance of your study. Citing other studies that suggest why your study is important or why your educational program would be of societal value allows you to build a strong case in the significance section of the proposal. It is not redundant to cite certain works in more than one place, although in the literature review section, a more thorough discussion is usually required.

The third reason for conducting a literature review is that it demonstrates the relevance of your topic to the body of knowledge that exists in a particular area. Thus, it provides the scientific or empirical evidence for pursuing your idea.

Fourth, the literature reviews help to identify and describe the theoretical foundation of your project. Showing relevance allows you to claim that your study or your program will add to the organized knowledge in a field, and identification of the theoretical framework will show that your project is grounded in a solid foundation.

Finally, the literature review will help determine the best strategy to use in carrying out your project. Often, reviewing approaches that other investigators have taken can suggest how best to pose a research query and develop the specific design, measures, and set of procedures.

There are several different ways to approach a literature review. Although we recommend the following approach, there is no one best way. It is often a matter of personal style and comfort (Findley, 1989).

Start by conducting a literature search in your library for articles or research studies that are directly related to the major focus of your project. A good rule of thumb is to review literature that has been published within the past five years unless there is an older "classic" article. Also, be sure to search the literature in fields other than yours. Review the abstracts of the articles and organize them into four categories:

1. highly relevant and absolutely essential for you to read for your proposal

2. somewhat relevant and will probably be used

3. relevant and you might use

4. not relevant

Begin with the most relevant articles and critically review them. Write down a very brief description of the article or study. If it is a research article, write a four to five sentence introduction in which you identify what was studied, how it was studied, what was found, and what conclusions were drawn. Also, discuss any recommendations for future research in these articles which support your proposed study. If it is not a research article, briefly summarize the major points of the article that are related to your topic. Once you have reviewed the articles in the "most relevant" category, do the same with the articles in the "relevant" category. If the conclusions and/or findings of the articles in these two categories are similar, it is probably time to stop searching for new articles.

There are at least two ways to organize the literature review. One approach is to present articles chronologically, with the oldest articles first, to provide a historical perspective. Another approach is to group articles according to common themes that are relevant to your topic. Let's take the educational project, discussed earlier, on providing care to individuals who are homeless. One strategy for reviewing and categorizing the related literature is to identify articles or studies that:

1. identify national and local statistics about the number of individuals who are homeless

2. contain demographic data about the homeless population

3. describe the health care needs of those who are homeless

4. describe problems faced by those who are homeless in accessing the health care system

5. discuss the need for new models in delivering health care

6. discuss the importance of interdisciplinary, community-based health care

7. discuss the role of each of the nursing and allied health professions in meeting the health care needs of those who are homeless

To cover the above points, you would need to search a number of different bodies of literature. These may include studies on team building and collaboration, epidemiological, social work and sociological research on homeless populations, government research reports, and related literature in each of the health professions that are participating in the project.

In reviewing the literature, it is important to consider resources outside your own field or profession and to obtain sources in which the original work in an area is conducted. For example, if you are planning to study a management issue, it is important to search the management literature; if you are studying an educational issue, be sure to examine articles from the educational journals that are pertinent to the topic.

If your topic area has not been studied or written about extensively, your review may be relatively brief. You then need to demonstrate that your topic is significant and cite the lack of research as one reason for conducting your study. A critical point to remember in writing a literature review is that the information you use and report must be from primary sources. A primary source is the original article from which this information is reported. It is almost never appropriate to discuss a research article that is described or presented in an article by an author who did not conduct or report on the original study.

At the conclusion of the literature review, provide a summary that reflects a synthesis and analysis of the articles. In this concluding section, you should discuss the way the cited literature supports your background, significance, research question, hypotheses, and/or design. Also, identify the gaps in knowledge and the way in which your study or educational program systematically contributes to knowledge building and addresses these gaps. Once you write this section of the proposal, ask yourself the following questions.

BOX 5-7

SELF-STUDY QUESTIONS

1. Does the literature review present important background information about the proposal topic?
2. Does the literature review critically evaluate and synthesize existing knowledge?
3. Are the identified gaps in knowledge addressed by this study or program?
4. Does the review provide a basis of support for the hypotheses and/or research question?
5. Has the need for the proposed study been documented?
6. Does the literature review appear complete and up-to-date?
7. Is the literature review logically and systematically developed and presented?

g. *Methodology/research or educational plan*—If you are writing a proposal for a training or demonstration grant, this section will contain a detailed description of each step you plan to take to carry out your project. This plan of operation must be carefully developed and comprehensive. In this section, you are answering the question, "How will you carry out the project?" Thus, organize your description in a step-by-step logical manner and explain in detail the activities you will implement to accomplish each objective. The review panel will want to examine the details of your plans, such as course development and student recruitment. They will also evaluate whether you are proposing a logical sequence of courses or training experiences and/or how your plan complements, improves, or extends existing programs. Consider using flow charts and tables to describe the curriculum or project design. Graphic displays provide a concise visual summary of your written material and reinforce the major points in the narrative.

If you propose a research study, the methodology section is critical. Each aspect of the research design must be described in detail. As with an education program, you must explain in a logical way, the specific procedures for recruiting study participants, collecting data and analyzing the results. Also you need to provide a justification for each methodological decision, procedure, design elements and analytic plan. Key aspects of your research design that you must present are outlined in Box 5-8.

BOX 5-8

SUGGESTED SUBSECTIONS OF RESEARCH METHODOLOGY

1. Overview of research design
2. Sample description and selection
   a. Inclusion and exclusion criteria
   b. Recruitment plan
3. Procedures, materials, and data collection
4. Human Subjects
5. Study validity and reliability
6. Assumptions and study limitations
7. Time table of key research activities
8. Statistical analysis for each study aim

It is important to consult with a statistician in developing your specific aims, study procedures and analytic design. A statistician may also agree to assist in writing this section of the proposal in exchange for a paid consultancy to the project if it is funded.

Common mistakes made by applicants in this section include providing an inadequate justification for why a particular procedure or approach is chosen, poor integration of ideas, incorrect or inappropriate statistical or research design, and lack of sufficient detail about the recruitment and general research procedures. These mistakes can be avoided by carefully planning each aspect of the design, by developing drafts that can be reviewed by another researcher or statistical consultant, and by pilot testing different aspects of the design (e.g., to determine feasibility of recruitment plan).

Be aware of a "fatal flaw." A fatal flaw represents a fundamental problem in the research design that cannot be remedied by simple alterations in the proposal. A design flaw requires a rethinking and restructuring of the entire project. Box 5-9 presents a comment from a review panel that reflects a fatal flaw in a proposal.

BOX 5-9

EXAMPLE OF A FATAL FLAW

It is difficult to see how this research study, with its cohort design, will adequately test the outcomes of the proposed intervention as it is currently conceptualized. Since random assignment of patients to experimental and control groups would compromise patient treatment plans at this facility, it would be unethical and not feasible to do so. However, without randomization, study outcomes cannot be interpreted in any meaningful way, nor can treatment effectiveness be determined.

Let's examine each subsection of the methodology section in more detail. Keep in mind that there is not a specific order in which each one of the subsections below should be presented. Rather, your research plan must be presented in a logical order and reflect an integration of ideas.

    a. *Research design*—The research design of a study is the "blueprint" or plan that describes the way in which the study will be organized, the variables that will be measured and the data collection and analytic procedures that will be followed (DePoy & Gitlin, 1998). Each component of the research design must be presented clearly and concisely. A justification for each aspect of the design should also be provided.

Begin the research design section with an overview, in which you identify and label your design (e.g., a two-group randomized experimental design; retrospective chart review; 2 X 2 X 2 factorial design) and explain why the design is appropriate to control variance and threats to validity.

Second, specify the major elements of the design, such as the independent and dependent variables, the sampling frame, sample size and selection procedures, and the number of testing occasions that are planned. It is important to be very specific in your description. For example, when specifying the independent and dependent variables, explain how each is related in the study (e.g., causal, explanatory, mediator, predictor). Two examples of design statements are presented in Boxes 5-10 and 5-11.

BOX 5-10

DESIGN STATEMENT #1

This study is designed to evaluate the level of knowledge of case managers in homeless shelters regarding the health care needs of their clients. A descriptive survey design using a stratified random sample is proposed by which 100 case managers from 30 homeless shelters in the City of Philadelphia will be randomly selected to complete a questionnaire designed to assess four areas of knowledge. These are: oral hygiene, mental health, drug and alcohol problems, and basic hygiene. The survey will contain demographic information, multiple choice questions that tap knowledge of signs and symptoms of each problem, and open-ended questions that ask respondents to describe their approach to dealing with each problem.

BOX 5-11

DESIGN STATEMENT #2

The research design chosen for this study is a randomized two group experimental design to test the effectiveness of a home-based intervention for families caring for individuals with dementia. The study involves 250 caregivers who are assigned to either a treatment or control group. Study participants in the treatment group receive five home visits by an occupational therapist, whereas those in the control group do not receive any grant-supported services. A three month post-test will evaluate the immediate effect of the intervention on caregiver skill acquisition, use of environmental modifications, and level of burden. Six- and twelve-month follow-up interviews will assess long-term effects of the intervention.

After completing the draft of a design statement, ask yourself the following questions.

BOX 5-12

SELF-STUDY QUESTIONS

1. Is the research design appropriate to study the research problem?
2. Does the research design control for extraneous variables and threats to validity?

---

b. *Sample description and selection*—In this subsection the characteristics of the sample and the procedures by which study participants will be selected are described. Five basic points should be covered.

1. Describe the criteria that will be used to select study participants. This involves listing the specific criteria for inclusion and exclusion of study participants and the reason or justification for each of these criteria.

2. Describe the anticipated characteristics of the study participants and the extent to which these are representative of the population to which you plan to generalize the study findings. In discussing the sample characteristics, include a description of age, gender, race, ethnicity, and health status.

3. Describe the procedures you will use for recruiting the sample.

4. Discuss the sample size and the justification for its adequacy using power analysis, if appropriate.

5. Provide evidence of the feasibility of obtaining the required sample.

BOX 5-13

EXAMPLE OF SAMPLE DESCRIPTION #1

Participants in this study will comprise a convenience sample of 250 caregivers living with and caring for a family member with moderate dementia. Caregivers whose recipient has Parkinson's disease or who is on experimental medication will be excluded from the study. The sample size of 250 is adequate to detect outcomes and is based on a power analysis, with power set at .80, alpha at .05, and an anticipated moderate effect size. No difficulty is anticipated in obtaining a sample of 250 caregivers since previous analysis of the five dementia clinics participating in this study report an average of 30 new clients per month for the past two years who fit the study criteria.

BOX 5-14

EXAMPLE OF SAMPLE DESCRIPTION #2

This study will be comprised of a convenience sample of 20 HIV-positive Hispanic men attending an AIDS support group who volunteer to participate in the study. Criteria for eligibility include evidence of an HIV positive test and a 90% attendance record at support group meetings for the previous six months.

Currently, there is an active pool of 50 men who have been tested as HIV positive. Subject recruitment will occur by two methods. The first method will entail a letter to each active participant which describes the purpose of the study and invites participation. The second method will entail an explanation of the study by the principal investigator at regular meetings of the support group. Those who agree to participate will be interviewed to determine their eligibility.

Once you have a draft of this section, ask yourself these questions.

BOX 5-15

SELF-STUDY QUESTIONS

1. Is the sample representative of the population of interest?
2. Is the sample size adequate?
3. Is the description of how the sample will be derived clearly stated?
4. Is the sampling procedure appropriate (free of sampling error or bias)?
5. Are the procedures described in sufficient detail to allow for replication?
6. Is the assignment of subject to groups appropriate and adequately described?

c. *Procedures, materials, or data collection instruments*—This subsection should include a discussion of the procedures you will follow in collecting data and the instruments you will use.

First, provide a detailed description of the procedures you intend to implement for data collection. Think about what you need to do if your grant is funded and describe these steps in detail. Boxes 5-16 and 5-17 provide examples of discussions about procedures.

BOX 5-16

EXAMPLES OF PROCEDURE DISCUSSIONS

#1

Following notification of grant approval and funding, a letter will be mailed to administrators of participating nursing homes. This letter will explain the purpose of the study and its procedures and the importance of participation of the nursing assistants. The letter will be followed by a telephone call to the administrator to determine an appropriate time for a 20-minute telephone survey with each nursing assistant. Each participating nursing home will be requested to provide a quiet office setting from which the nursing assistant can participate in the telephone survey.

#2

Cultures will be obtained from 20 HIV-positive patients and identified and quantified on a weekly basis until the infection has been controlled. Thereafter, cultures will be taken monthly for a maximum of 12 months. Treatments will be administered to control the clinical signs and symptoms.

Second, discuss the materials that are necessary or the data collection instruments that will be used for the study. In describing a data collection instrument, discuss its domains (e.g., demographic information, job satisfaction, psychological stress), the measurement level of a scale, and its validity and reliability for the specific group of subjects included in your study. If you intend to design a data collection instrument, discuss a plan for examining its reliability and obtaining at least face or content validity. Important aspects to discuss are noted in Box 5-17.

BOX 5-17

DATA COLLECTION INSTRUMENTS AND STRATEGIES

a. Describe your data collection instruments.
   - What is their published reliability?
   - What is their published validity?
   - How extensively are they used in other research?
   - Why did you choose these particular instruments?

b. Describe your data collection strategies.
   - How will you collect the data?
   - If you interview subjects, what procedures will you use?

BOX 5-18

EXAMPLE OF A DISCUSSION OF INSTRUMENTATION

The telephone survey will be developed by the investigators and consist of three primary domains: demographic and background information, items which assess knowledge of oral pathology in the elderly; and a case vignette with questions to determine the ability to recognize signs and symptoms of disease. The survey will be reviewed by five individuals with expertise in oral health care of the elderly. This panel of experts will independently review the survey for its content validity. Modifications to the survey instrument will be made based on the panel's review and the survey will be pilot tested with five nursing assistants.

d. *Human subjects*—This subsection provides a discussion of the protection of human subjects. The discussion should include: a) your plans to assure confidentiality of the information or data that you obtain from human subjects, b) how consent from study participants will be obtained, c) the potential benefits and risks for a subject associated with participation, and d) the risk benefit ratio (see also the discussion on the IRB in chapter 4).

BOX 5-19

EXAMPLE OF DISCUSSION OF HUMAN SUBJECTS

This research is descriptive and involves a telephone survey. Participation in the study will be voluntary and by responding to the telephone survey, respondents will be giving their informed consent to participate. Subject confidentiality will be assured by the use of identification numbers on data sheets. Subject names and other identifying information will be kept in a locked filing cabinet in the office of the investigator and will be separate from the information provided by subjects in response to the survey questions. Information will be reported in aggregate form only and no participant will be identified.

There are no potential risks to participants. There are no direct personal benefits except for personal satisfaction obtained in participating in research and contributing to building a body of knowledge.

---

e. *Validity and reliability*—In this subsection you need to address both the validity and reliability of your design. Validity refers to whether a design and its procedures are appropriate and will yield information to answer the research question. You need to explain the specific procedures that will assure that your approach is the appropriate way to answer your research question. For example, if your purpose is to demonstrate causality, you would use an experimental design and would need to discuss why the particular design you chose is most appropriate.

You also need to consider the reliability of your approach to data collection and analysis. Clearly describe the specific design features you have established that will assure consistency of procedures in such a way that another investigator could replicate your study. For example, let's say you are obtaining cultures of oral lesions. Discuss the exact procedures you plan to implement to assure that all investigators take cultures from the correct lesion and use the same technique.

f. *Assumptions and limitations*—In this subsection, your discussion would focus on the specific limitations of your design. Almost every study has some limitations either based on features inherent in the design or in its application to your particular situation. Think about these limitations and how they may introduce possible sources of bias. For example, let's say you are conducting a Delphi study. A limitation of this technique is the possibility that some respondents may discuss their opinions with others who they know are also participating in the study. This is a limitation that may have consequences for your findings. Thus, you should identify this limitation and discuss the way you plan to address it.

g. *Time table*—Base your start-up date and the length of time that will be required to accomplish the major activities of your study on the earliest possible funding date for your proposal. Then provide a table which summarizes each major activity and the time frame for its completion.

Here are two examples of how you might present this material.

BOX 5-20

EXAMPLE #1 OF TIME TABLE

ACTIVITY	TIME FRAME
1. Questionnaire development	Months 1–3
2. Pilot testing of instruments	Months 4
3. Subject recruitment	Months 5–8
4. Subject interviewing	Months 5–10
5. Data entry, data cleaning	Months 10–12
6. Data analysis	Months 12–15
7. Report generation	Months 15–18

BOX 5-21

EXAMPLE #2 OF TIME TABLE

ACTIVITY	July	Aug.	Sept.	Oct.	Nov.	Dec.	Jan.	Feb.
Instrument development	X	X						
Pilot test of protocol			X					
Sample selection			X					
Mail survey				X				
Reminder notice					X			
Second reminder notice						X		
Data entry and analysis						X	X	
Report writing and dissemination								X

BOX 5-22

SELF-STUDY QUESTIONS FOR METHODS AND
MATERIALS SECTION

1. Is the design appropriate for the research ques-
    tion and logically developed?
2. Are the measures selected adequate and has
    reliability and validity been addressed?
3. Is there a timetable of major activities that
    accurately reflects the requirements of the
    study design and provides an adequate time
    frame for each activity?

Once you have completed a draft of this section, consider
these questions as a way of reflecting upon your proposal.

h. *Statistical analysis*—This section involves a discussion of
    your analytic strategy and the statistical tests you plan to
    use. In your discussion, it is helpful to restate the specific
    aims and hypotheses of your study and then identify the
    statistical tests that will be used to address each
    aim/hypothesis. Also, provide a brief rationale for your
    choice of tests and the significance level that will be used
    to determine statistical significance.

    Be sure that the analyses you select fit the measurement
    level of your data. For example, if your data is categorical
    or ordinal, then a descriptive and non-parametric statisti-
    cal approach should be used. Your primary method of
    presentation would be frequency tables involving distribu-
    tion of percentages. You may need to consult with a statis-
    tician to determine the best analytic approach for your
    study. Keep in mind that the analyses you choose are an
    extension of your study design and must answer the
    research question. Box 5-23 provides two examples of
    discussions of statistical designs.

BOX 5-23

EXAMPLE #1 OF A DISCUSSION OF STATISTICAL ANALYSIS

The major hypothesis which will be tested in this study is that students who participate in a computer assistive learning experience will demonstrate greater knowledge of oral pathology and greater satisfaction with their educational experience than students who take a traditional didactic course. Analysis of covariance (ANCOVA) will be used as the primary statistical test to evaluate the experimental effect on the two dependent variables (knowledge of oral pathology and student satisfaction). ANCOVA is the statistical test typically used in a two-group experimental design involving pre- and post-test data.

Also, demographic data obtained from this study will be tabulated using crosstab frequency distributions and measures of central tendency. All tests of significance will be reported at the .05 level.

EXAMPLE #2 OF A DISCUSSION OF STATISTICAL ANALYSIS

A combination of statistical methods will be used to compare the characteristics of dental hygienists who participate in the mail survey questionnaire. Analysis of categorical variables will involve crosstab frequency distributions with chi-square statistics. Comparisons of the two groups (novice and experienced dental hygienists) on continuous variables will be based on analysis of variance (ANOVA). Significant ANOVAs will be followed up with Tukey's HSD (Honestly Significant Difference) test for multiple comparisons. To determine statistical significance, alpha will be set at .01 to control for Type I error and all statistical tests will be based on a two-tailed distribution.

Once you complete your discussion of the statistical analysis, ask yourself the following self-study questions as a check to see that you have included all of the appropriate material.

BOX 5-24

SELF-STUDY QUESTIONS FOR STATISTICAL SECTION

1. Are the statistical analyses appropriate to answer my research question and test the proposed hypotheses?
2. Are the statistical analyses appropriate for the measurement level of the data which will be collected?

i. *Dissemination plan*—Some agencies seek to assure that the results of a successful project they have funded have a wide impact. From their perspective, it makes little sense to fund a project if only a few people will benefit. Therefore, agencies may require that you present a systematic plan for disseminating the results of your project. Two important and commonly accepted ways to disseminate project results is through presentations at national, scientific, and professional meetings, and publication in professional journals. You should also develop other creative or innovative ways to assure a wide distribution of your findings. These may include the development and distribution of instructional manuals, conducting workshops or continuing education programs, or implementing innovative ways to reach consumers as well as professional groups.

j. *Plan of management*—In this section, you must answer the question as to why you are the most appropriate person to carry out this project. Although you may have a wonderful idea, you must also assure an agency that you have the necessary expertise and resources to accomplish the program goals efficiently. You will need to demonstrate that you have a clear, logical, and efficient plan of management that will be executed by a project team comprised of well-qualified people at an institution that can provide the necessary support and resources. A clear description of the organizational and management structure will answer the first part of this question. In your management plan, you should discuss in detail the roles and responsibilities of key personnel, the amount of time each person will work on the project, and the time frame in which each project task will be carried out. Agencies usually want to see this information organized in the form of a time line or a detailed Grant chart of major activities.

One approach to writing this section is to visualize that you have already been funded. Think about the steps you would have to take to carry out your plan if you were to start tomorrow. Who would you need to hire? What contacts would be important? What resources would you need? Logically and rationally think through your plan before you write the section. This may raise critical points of weakness in your research or curriculum design, or it may highlight limitations in institutional resources that you will need to address or offset.

k. *Investigative team credentials*—This section also helps answer the question about your qualifications to carry out the project. Review your plan to determine the special skills that are necessary to carry out each step of the project and carefully select team members with this expertise. For example, if you are proposing a study that requires a repeated measures design or statistical modeling techniques, make sure you have a statistician on your team with expertise in these specific analytic strategies. If your study uses naturalistic inquiry, you will need to assure that a member of your team is an expert in qualitative methodologies and software programs. In writing an educational grant, make sure you are working with someone who has curriculum development skills. Select individuals with complementary experience and credentials. For example, in an educational grant, you might need two people, one with curriculum development skills and one with experience in curriculum evaluation.

For some grant applications, you will need to include a brief descriptive paragraph highlighting the qualifications of each member. Emphasize their past experience, publications, or presentations that show expertise in the topic of the project. You should also cite funding for other projects, either from sources that are external to your institution or from your institution, which you or other members have received. Sometimes offices held in professional organizations, teaching or consulting experiences provide additional credibility and demonstrate that you have the necessary background to implement the project successfully.

l. *Institutional qualifications*—Just as you need to develop a qualified team, your institution needs to have the resources to assist and support you in carrying out your project. You will need to include a concise description of your institutional resources and its qualifications. For example, has your institution acquired a significant amount of external funding? Does it have a comprehensive library, a learning resource center, or an active research administration office? What computer facilities are available for your use?

m. *Budget*—This section addresses questions regarding the cost of your project and why it will cost what it does. You need to prepare a budget that is not inflated or wasteful and still sufficient to accomplish all your activities. Do not try to "pad" your budget by inflating costs or adding unnecessary expenses. Also do not underestimate what it will cost you to carry out the study or educational program. The best rule of thumb is to develop a budget that accurately reflects the cost of the activities you are proposing. Most institutions have budget offices or offices of research administration that can help you prepare this budget.

You will also be required to justify each expense in a budget justification section following the actual budget. In this section describe what each item will be used for and why it is necessary for your project. We discuss budget preparation in more detail in chapter 6.

n. *References*—As in all scientific work, a reference list of your primary sources of information is required. If the agency does not specify a reference style, then use the style specified by the American Psychological Association (APA). In all cases, be sure to be consistent in the presentation of references. Also, be sure to check the instructions to determine if there is a page limitation for this section. For an NIH grant, using the PHS 398 forms no page limitation for references are specified, but applicants are urged to include only those cited and most pertinent to the grant.

o. *Appendix material*—The appendices usually include information that supplements the narrative. For example, appendix material may include the complete curriculum vitae of key members of the project team, sample questionnaires or evaluation instruments, pertinent articles that you have authored which relate to the project, curriculum materials, and, most importantly, letters of support from consultants, leaders in your profession, or your senators and congressmen.

SUMMARY

This chapter describes the basic elements of the grant application. Although each agency structures their calls for proposals differently, there are sections that are commonly required. In this chapter we identified the content of each section and ways to approach its writing. Four major points have been made:

1. A proposal is simply a document in which you propose to carry out an idea. Its main purpose is to convince a funding agency that it should provide money to support the implementation of your idea.

2. The sections of a proposal can be thought of as answers to a series of questions. These questions are: What is your project about? Why is it important? What will you plan to do? How will you do it? What will it cost and why? Why are you the best one to do it?

3. Funding agencies are interested in receiving the best possible proposals. Therefore, they will usually provide detailed instructions regarding what should be included in your proposal and criteria upon which it will be evaluated.

4. The instructions provided by the agency provide a guideline as to how to structure the components of the proposal. Therefore, the instructions should be carefully read, reread, and reread.

Chapter 6

Preparing A Budget

- Information Required for Developing a Budget
- Basic Components of a Budget
- Budget Justification
- NIH Modular Format

6.1 INFORMATION REQUIRED FOR DEVELOPING A BUDGET

There are three important considerations in preparing a budget for a grant application: 1) the policies and requirements of the agency from which grant funds are being sought, 2) the policies and requirements of your institution, and 3) the resources needed and costs associated with each task of the project.

Agency requirements: Prior to developing a proposal budget, it is important to learn the types of activities and budgetary categories that an agency will fund as part of the grant program as well as the way in which you will be expected to manage the budget if you should receive the award. Table 6-1 outlines the key questions you need to ask a project officer or find answers to in the application kit before developing the budget.

TABLE 6-1   Agency Budget Questions

I. Questions regarding the competition

- What is the projected average cost of a project that will be funded in this competition?
- What is the maximum amount of money that can be requested and does this reflect direct and facilities and administrative (F&A) or indirect costs?
- What is the allowable F & A cost recovery rate that can be requested?
- What are the allowable budget costs for each budget category?

II. Questions regarding budget management

- Can funds be carried over from one project year to the next?
- Is there level funding or can variable amounts or cost of living increases be requested each project year?
- Are no-cost extensions granted at the end of the project period to carry out any uncompleted grant activities?

First, it is important to learn if there is a limit imposed on the amount of money that can be requested and whether that limit includes direct and F&A costs. Box 6-1 contains an example of how this information may be provided in a request for applications (RFA).

BOX 6-1

EXAMPLE OF BUDGET SPECIFICATIONS PROVIDED IN AN RFA

Approximately $2.0 million is projected to be available in FY '03 to fund six to nine grants. The amount of funding actually available may vary and is subject to change. New grant awards will not exceed $300,000 per year (including both direct and F&A costs). Grant applications that exceed the $300,000 per year cap will be returned to the investigator as non-responsive.

Although an agency may not specify the amount of funds that an investigator can request in a particular competition, it may indicate the anticipated average award. This information is important because it lets you know the scope of the projects the agency is seeking to support. This information will help guide your decisions about the number of activities you should propose as well as the upper limits of your budget. For example, let's say an agency anticipates granting an average of $150,000 per project and this amount includes both the direct costs of the project and the allowable F & A costs. An application in which the budget significantly exceeds that amount may be evaluated poorly or, if funded, the grant budget may be reduced to fit the agency's expectations. In some cases, as noted in Box 6-1, the agency may impose a strict upper limit that it will fund. Applications that exceed that limit will be returned to the investigator without being reviewed.

Each agency has its own rules about expenses that are allowed and those that are not. These rules may also differ for each competition that is sponsored by the same agency. For example, a number of professional associations sponsor competitions that do not support salary for the investigator, graduate student tuition, stipends, travel to professional meetings, or equipment costs. Many requests for applications that are issued by federal agencies do not support costs associated with renovation of existing facilities, equipment, or direct patient care. Also, the NIH imposes a cap on the total salary that can be offset in their applications. Therefore, it is very important for you to learn what expenses are allowed.

The facilities and administrative cost recovery rate (also referred to as indirect costs) differ depending on the agency and the type of competition. For example, some foundations allow an 8% or 10% F&A cost rate, while others will not allow any F&A charges. Some agencies at the federal level have a set rate. If this rate is not published in the application kit, you should ask a program officer. The NIH negotiates a rate with each institution. This information should be available from your Office of Research Administration. The application kit also specifies any other budget restrictions or guidelines that apply to a competition. Conversely, some competitions specify the types of costs that are expected. For example, some competitions require that the principal investigator commit a certain level of effort on the proposed project.

It is also important to know an agency's rules for managing grant budgets. These rules will differ among agencies and competitions and may determine the way in which you develop a budget.

For example, some agencies allow an investigator to use funds that are not spent in one project year in the subsequent budget year. These are called "carry forward" or "carry over" funds. However, some agencies do not allow funds to be carried over. That is, if you do not spend funds allocated for one project year, then these are lost to you. This has implications for planning activities of a project. If certain activities are not accomplished before the end of the budget year, then there will be no funds to carry them out at a later time. We discuss ways to manage budgets and carry over funds in more detail in chapter 13.

It is also important to learn whether a funding agency allows varying budgeted amounts each year or yearly increases due to salary and cost of living adjustments, or whether there is what is called "level funding." If an agency enforces level funding, then the total budget request for the first year is the amount that will be awarded in each subsequent year of the project.

Level funding has important implications for the way in which you plan the flow of project activities. With level funding it is essential to evenly distribute activities over each budget year of the project. For example, let's say you are planning an education program for students in allied health. In your first year, you propose a long start-up period involving significant coordination and planning activities. Your budget will, therefore, be modest since these are relatively inexpensive activities. In your second year you plan to actively recruit 40 students, hire three new faculty members and two new clinical supervisors to instruct in the courses that are developed. In this year your budget will necessarily increase significantly from the first year. If the agency allows budgets to fluctuate from year to year then there are no difficulties with this project plan. However, if level funding is required by the agency, then it would be difficult to carry out the project plan since you would only receive the same level of funding each project year.

Most agencies allow what are referred to as "no cost extensions." A "no cost extension" enables an investigator to extend grant activities beyond its funded period by using unspent funds from the final year to complete the project activities in the following year. This flexibility is important especially in research grants where many activities, such as subject recruitment and interviewing, can be delayed due to circumstances that are beyond the control of the investigator. Although it is important to know whether an agency allows a no-cost extension, this should have no immediate effect on how you plan the budget for your proposal submission. Nevertheless, it is essential to understand an agency's budgetary expectations and rules for management and thus it is best to contact a program officer to clarify these rules that are often unwritten.

Institutional policies: A second important consideration in preparing a grant budget is the specific requirements of your institution. For example, you need to conform to your institution's personnel salary scale, and apply the institutional rate for fringe benefits and F&A cost recovery. Table 6-2 lists the six basic questions to ask an official in your institution to help you prepare a grant budget. Depending upon the organizational structure of your institution, you can obtain this information from either the office of the controller, office of the budget administrator, office of research administration, or the office of sponsored programs.

TABLE 6-2   Institutional-Related Budget Considerations

- What is the institution's fringe benefit rate?
- What is the institution's projected yearly percent merit or inflationary salary increase?
- What is the institution's F&A cost recovery rate?
- What is the salary range for key personnel who need to be hired?
- What is the institution's rate for car travel reimbursement?
- What will the institution permit as in-kind contributions?

Most institutions develop a set of procedures for reviewing the budgets of proposals to assure that it conforms to their requirements. Some large universities might even develop the budget for an investigator.

Project cost considerations: Finally, in developing a budget for a proposal, you need to carefully estimate the resources required to complete each project task, and develop a realistic budget that accurately reflects the cost of each task. That is, your budget should reflect what you actually need and not what would be nice to have. It should also use and build upon the resources of your institution. For example, although it would be nice to have a full-time secretary on your project, most do not require this level of support. Therefore, it would be inappropriate to request a 100%

secretarial position when only a 30% effort is actually required. By building on the resources at your institution, you may be able to increase the time of a part-time secretary, or renegotiate the role of a full-time secretary so that 30% of his or her effort will be devoted to your project.

Budget considerations will also influence the design of the project and its scope. The budget you request should accurately reflect the costs associated with each project activity. Therefore, you need to think about the budget as you develop your program to assure that you can accomplish your project with the amount of money which will be available to you.

As you develop the budget, ask yourself the questions in Table 6-3 as a guide.

TABLE 6-3   Self-Study Questions for Budget Development

1. Is my budget practical and realistic for the tasks I plan to accomplish?
2. Is my budget appropriate for the tasks I need to accomplish, my level of resources, and the costs allowable by the agency?
3. Are the grant funds I am requesting sufficient to offset the costs of my project?
4. Is my budget comprehensive in that it covers all costs associated with the implementation of my project?

6.2 BASIC COMPONENTS OF A BUDGET

There are usually three major components of a proposal budget: 1) direct costs, 2) F&A cost allowance, and 3) institutional commitments. Let's look at each of these components and discuss strategies for developing a budget.

Direct costs: Direct costs are those expenses that are necessary to carry out your project. The following eight budget categories are required by most federal agencies and foundations.

1. *Personnel*—This category refers to the salary and fringe benefit support that is requested for each member of the project team. The project team usually includes individuals such as the principal investigator, project director or coordinator, interviewers, research assistants, statisticians, and secretaries. Starting with the principal investigator, list the names and identify the roles of all the people who will be involved on the project during the budget period. In this section, list only those who are current employees of your institution or who will be hired by the institution to work on the grant. To determine the cost of these salaries, first estimate the amount of time each person will spend on the project. Usually, this is calculated as a percentage of a person's full-time job commitment. Next, multiply this percentage by an individual's annual base salary. If the person is on a nine- or 10-month employment contract and is asked to work on the grant during the summer months, a separate calculation for the summer salary will be required. The next step is to compute the cost of fringe benefits that are attributable to this salary. This rate is determined by your institution. These two figures are then added to determine the person's salary paid for by the grant. Box 6-2 provides an example of how to compute a salary line.

   Similar calculations are made for all members of the project team.

2. *Consultants*—Consultants are those individuals who are not university employees but who you plan to hire to carry out discrete activities on your project. For example, on a research grant you might require the assistance of a cost analyst to guide cost effectiveness analyses you plan to conduct. On a training grant you may need to consult with an individual who is a recognized expert on the curriculum content of your program. You need to negotiate with the consultant the amount of his/her compensation and report it in this non-salary section of the budget. Fringe benefits are not calculated for consultant fees. However, consultants may request an amount that may include their own institution's fringe benefit rate.

BOX 6-2

EXAMPLE OF SALARY CALCULATION

Dr. J. is an assistant professor of physical therapy with a 10-month salary of $55,000. She has been included as a faculty member in an application for a training grant that the department is submitting. The principal investigator, Dr. M., has determined that she needs 15% of Dr. J.'s time during the academic year, and 100% of her time for one month during the summer. The university fringe benefit rate is 26.5%. Dr. M. computes her salary line in the following manner. First, she takes 15% of $55,000 = $8,250. This is Dr. J.'s salary covered by the grant during the academic year. Dr. M. then computes her benefit allowance by multiplying $8,250 by 26.5%, or $2,186. This is the fringe benefit cost rounded to the nearest whole dollar. The fringe benefit cost is added to the salary ($8,250 + $2,186 = $10,436), to determine the total grant contribution to Dr. J.'s salary during the academic year. Dr. J. will also work for one month during the summer, and a separate calculation needs to be made for this month. Since Dr. J. is on a 10-month contract, her monthly salary is $5,500 ($55,000 x 10%), and her fringe benefit rate will be $1,458 (26.5% x $5,500). Therefore, her summer compensation will be $6,958 ($5,500 + $1,458), and her total grant supported salary will be $17,394 ($10, 436 + $6,958).

---

3. *Equipment*—Items such as furniture or equipment that have a usable life of two or more years and cost over $500.00 are reported in this section. Computers, slide projectors, fax machines, or special laboratory equipment are the types of equipment that fall into this category. The full cost of these should be reported. A word of caution is in order here. You should only request funding for equipment that is essential and directly related to your project and not already available at your institution.

Since equipment may last longer than the life of your grant, review panels and funding agencies examine this category closely to assure the appropriateness of your request and that you are not "padding your budget" to purchase items that may be used for other projects and persons in your department. For example, at one point personal computers were not common in faculty offices or laboratories and many investigators needed to purchase them with grant funds. Today, the purchase of personal computers for employees is usually considered the responsibility of the institution and funding agencies are rarely willing to support this purchase. Money for items such as slide projectors is almost never approved since agencies also consider the purchase of such equipment as the responsibility of your institution. In order to obtain approval for the purchase of durable, fixed equipment, you must provide a strong justification for its importance to your project and a rationale as to why the funding agency, rather than your institution should support the cost.

4. *Supplies*—These include daily office needs such as stationery, audiotapes, and specific laboratory supplies, such as reagents and chemicals, that are necessary for your project. However, federal agencies no longer approve the use of direct costs for general office supplies such as paper, pencils, computer disks. Often, there is no need to itemize supplies if your total request is less than $1,000.00. As with all proposed purchases, estimate as closely as you can the cost of all the materials you will need and ask for that amount with a justification for the expenditure.

5. *Trainee expenses*—This category is usually found only in applications for training grants. All costs related to individuals, usually students, who will be the recipients of the training provided by the grant, are included in this section. These include expenses such as tuition, stipends, travel, or other costs associated with supporting the participation of trainees in your project.

6. *Travel*—Travel expenses include costs of transportation, lodging, meals, meeting registration fees, and incidental expenses associated with travel by project personnel. Travel costs must be directly related to your project. Examples include attending a conference to present a

paper; meetings with other investigators to discuss your project; travel for advisory board members on your project; and costs associated with interviewing subjects. You should request only clearly justifiable travel expenses and provide an estimate of hotel and transportation costs. All travel by airline must be in economy class. Also, your institution most likely will use the government rate for reimbursing travel by car. The current government rate is $ .36 a mile, but inquire whether this rate is used by your institution. Also, since this rate frequently changes it is best to check with your research administration prior to developing your budget.

7. *Alterations and renovations*—In some cases, agencies will fund alterations or renovations to a physical space, which are necessary to implement your project. For example, if you are conducting a study of wheelchair access, you may be able to receive funding for renovations to install ramps or widen doorways to an area that study participants will need to use. Costs for space rental are usually not allowable since these costs are included in the F&A cost recovery rate that your institution is legally permitted to request. Some foundations provide support for major construction projects such as the erection of a building. However, these "bricks and mortar" projects are becoming less common. For most beginning investigators, alterations and renovations will not be relevant budget items.

8. *Consortium/contractual costs*—There are a variety of projects in which a consortium relationship is necessary: a school of allied health may want to collaborate with a school of education to conduct an educational training project; a department of laboratory sciences might want to work with an equipment company in a study of new technology; or a department of occupational therapy might want to develop an agreement with a rehabilitation hospital to study a particular therapeutic intervention. These types of arrangements require special agreements between the participating institutions.

The two most common arrangements are consortium and contractual agreements. In a consortium arrangement, both parties have responsibility for the scope of the entire project, although each will carry out different aspects.

However, one institution will be required to serve as the principal institution and oversee the receipt and disbursement of funds. Another approach would be to contract with another institution for specific services. In either case, each participating institution has their own rules regarding compensation of personnel, allowable costs, and overhead rates, and each will need to submit a separate budget. Most institutions have standard forms and specific procedures for entering into these types of agreements with outside agencies, so you will need to work closely with your Office of Research Administration to develop the appropriate legal documents.

If your institution is the lead or principal institution in a consortial or contractual arrangement, your organization will receive and disburse all funds. The participating institution will then periodically bill you for their services. Be certain that you have reached a clear agreement about the exact services that will be provided, how you will be notified of their completion, and a schedule of payments.

9. *"Other" expenses*—All expenses not specifically covered in other categories are reported in this section. These can include miscellaneous expenses such as lunch for an advisory board, long distance telephone costs, recruitment advertisement costs, or payments to subjects. For example, a project involving pediatric AIDS might include money in the budget for small gifts for the children as a way of encouraging participation and showing appreciation for a family's involvement.

Facilities and Administrative Costs: Since you will occupy institutional space and need administrative support (e.g., assistance from your office of research administration) for your project, government agencies and foundations have agreed to help defray associated costs. These include costs of building maintenance, utilities, insurance, and other general administrative expenses. An allowance for F&A or overhead expenses (also referred to as indirect costs) is based on a pre-negotiated percentage of certain direct costs of the grant. While F&A costs are included in your budget, they are used by your institution and are not available to you in carrying out your project, unless your institution has a policy for sharing some of these costs.

Overhead or indirect cost recovery rates for research grants vary widely and are officially negotiated between the university and a federal agency. For some agencies, such as the National Institutes of Health, the F&A rate may range from 50%-70% of modified total direct costs. This rate is added to the total budget for the grant when you submit your proposal. Other agencies, such as the U.S. Department of Education, do not have a standard negotiated rate for research projects. In this case, you need to propose an F&A cost recovery rate that is acceptable to your institution and which, when added to the direct costs, falls within the budget range stipulated by the agency.

Training grants have different F&A rates than research grants since most expenses are in the form of tuition and stipend payments to students. These and other related training activities do not directly use additional university resources. Therefore, the federal government uses a smaller F&A cost recovery rate that is usually 8%.

How do you calculate the F&A costs for your project? Not all expenses in your proposal can be used to compute your indirect cost recovery. This allowance is based on what is called modified direct cost. The general rule of thumb is that any expense in your grant that uses university facilities or resources is used to compute the modified direct costs. These include the expenses found in the following categories: personnel, travel, supplies, consultants, and "other." Equipment purchases, trainee expenses, and consortium and contractual costs over $500.00 are not allowable as part of the F&A cost base, since none of these uses the resources of your institution. However, for NIH grants, you are allowed to include the first $25,000 of consortium costs in calculating the indirect costs. In computing your F&A cost recovery, add the amounts in each of the allowable categories and multiply that amount by either 8% for a training grant or the negotiated rate of your institution for other types of projects. Simply add this amount to the total of the direct costs of your project to calculate the total costs for your project.

If your institution does not have a negotiated rate with the funding agency to which you are applying, you will need to discuss the most appropriate rate with your budget administrator or office of research administration and assure that the agency will accept this request as well. When you enter into an arrangement with another institution, their F&A cost recovery is included in the total amount of money that you agree to pay them, so separate calculations are not necessary.

Institutional commitments: An agency or a foundation may request, or in some instances require, that an institution contribute in some way to the financing of a project. Since cost-sharing commitments can have an effect on faculty and administrative workload, each institution has different policies related to the kinds and value of services that they are willing to commit. Cost sharing can be accomplished in several ways. First, an institution can contribute time for members on the project team. For example, if you estimate that a 40% effort is required by a member of your team, your institution may agree to donate 10% and ask the granting agency to pay 30%. Box 6-3 provides an example of how this might be done.

BOX 6-3

EXAMPLE OF INSTITUTIONAL COMMITMENT

Dr. K. is a member of a project team that involves a consortium arrangement between two universities. One of his administrative responsibilities is to encourage external relationships between his university and other agencies. Because the project requires a research or administrative liaison between the two universities, 10% of Dr. K.'s time is donated to the project for that purpose. Since this role is legitimately part of the grant activity and his daily responsibilities, it is an appropriate university contribution to the project.

Universities can also demonstrate commitment by waiving a portion of the F&A cost recovery allowance. If your university has a negotiated F&A cost rate of 60% with an agency such as NIH, you might request a lower rate, such as 50%, and show the difference (10%), as a university contribution. You should be aware that many universities would not agree to this option since it might jeopardize future F&A negotiations with NIH. However, if you are applying to an agency in which there is not a negotiated F&A cost rate, you could still use the 60% rate as a baseline to demonstrate an in-kind contribution.

A third way to demonstrate commitment is through the donation of supplies, mailing, phone, or duplicating expenses. For example, some universities have centralized mailing or purchasing systems that distribute costs for mailing and supplies throughout the university. For small mailings and limited supply purchases, the university might agree to share these costs with the granting agency.

These are all examples of legitimate cost sharing expenses. In developing a budget, be certain that your institution is agreeable to the in-kind commitments you include in the costs of your project. Most institutions are as concerned with the financial implications of a project as they are with its scientific integrity. Consequently, they typically have rules about what costs need to be covered in a grant budget. For example, some colleges and universities will interpret clerical or secretarial support, or basic office supplies as part of their F&A allowance. Others will allow you to request that the granting agency cover these expenses. Many institutions have an Office of Research Administration that is charged with overseeing all grants submitted at the institution and must approve all budget decisions. You need to check with this office prior to developing your budget. The staff will be familiar with the rules of your institution and assure that your budget is adequate.

Box 6-4 provides an example of a budget that shows how in-kind contributions might be presented in a budget.

6.3 BUDGET JUSTIFICATION

You are also required to provide a detailed justification for each expense you propose in your application. A budget justification involves a brief explanation and rationale for each line item in the budget. In writing the justification, start with "Personnel" and describe each person's roles and responsibilities on the project and provide a rationale for their percent effort. You will then need to systematically explain each line item of the budget and demonstrate how each cost is derived. Box 6-5 illustrates an excerpt from a budget justification for a training grant.

BOX 6-4

EXAMPLE OF A BUDGET CONTAINING IN-KIND CONTRIBUTIONS

Personnel

Position	% effort	Salary	Fringe (26.5)%	In-kind (10%)	Requested Amount
Investigator	40	14,400	3,816	6,092	18,216
Research Asst	10	1,800	477		2,277
Secretary	10	2,000	530		2,530
Subtotal:				6,092	23,025

Consultants

Survey design	10 hours	40/hr		400
Statistical support	5 hours	40/hr		200

Supplies

Envelopes	150
Printing and duplication	1,000

Staff Travel

Parking for meetings	100

Other

Data entry and computer use	500
Subtotal:	650

Total Project Costs	$31,467
Total Requested	$24,725
In-kind contribution	$ 6,742

BOX 6-5

EXAMPLE OF A BUDGET JUSTIFICATION FOR PERSONNEL

Personnel

Project Director—Dr. K.

Dr. K. will serve as the Project Manager on this Project. He will coordinate all project activities which include the following: convening of the Advisory Panel, overseeing the curriculum development activities, serving as liaison with the collaborating university, supervising graduate assistants, monitoring the grant budget, teaching in the newly designed courses, and participating in the dissemination activities. Dr. K. will devote 40% of his time to these efforts. The University will contribute 10% of his salary to this project. We are requesting 30% of Dr. K.'s salary from grant funds.

6.4 NIH MODULAR BUDGET FORMAT

It is worth noting that in 1999, the NIH instituted a new approach to reporting budget requests for grant applications in which the direct cost requirements in each year are $250,000 or less. For these applications, you must use what is referred to as the "modular format." This budget approach may be most relevant to new investigators who typically submit research grant applications with direct costs that are less than $250,000. However, this format must be used by any investigator who submits an application to the NIH when a modular format is required.

The modular format requires that the applicant request direct budget costs in $25,000 increments rather than showing details for each separate budget category. Using this approach, you typically request the same number of modules each year and show total direct costs on the PHS 398 form rather than providing detailed categorical budget information as discussed above. Let's say you develop a detailed budget and your total direct costs for the first year are $121,000. Using the modular budget format, you would request a total of $125,000. Likewise, let's say the second year direct costs are $123,500, you would request a total of $125,000. In year three, let's say the budget requirements increase to $140,000. You would then request $150,000 using the modular format.

A budget justification in the form of a narrative is still required. However, only specific information must be provided. Specifically, the justification must describe the per cent effort for key personnel, and consortium/contractual costs. Also, you must provide a rationale for yearly increments or decrements if the same number of modules is not requested each year. For example, in the scenario above, you would need to justify why the costs in your project increase by an additional $25,000 to $150,000 in the third year.

The modular budget format is part of a wider initiative of the NIH to streamline its procedures and refocus the efforts of investigators and review panels on the science of the application rather than budgetary and administrative details. This approach also streamlines the award process and eliminates renegotiations concerning budgetary details and the 25% rebudgeting requirement.

Although detailed information for each budget category is not submitted to NIH, it is still essential that you develop a detailed budget. A detailed budget will most likely be required by your institution and will also be necessary for you to effectively manage expenditures if you receive funding. Remember however, that even if you develop a detailed budget, do not submit this to the NIH if the modular format is required. Your application will be returned to you if you provide this excess information. Specific directions for modular budgeting can be found at http://grants.nih.gov/grants/funding/modular.htm.

SUMMARY

This chapter presented information that is necessary for preparing a grant budget. Six major points have been discussed:

1. In preparing a grant budget there are three considerations: the policies and requirements of the funding agency, the policies of your institution, and the costs associated with each project task.

2. Agencies provide information in the call for proposals regarding the number of grants expected to be funded and the estimated size of each grant award. This information should guide the development of a budget.

3. Each agency has their own rules about allowable and non-allowable expenses, the F&A cost recovery rate, and whether cost fluctuations from year to year. It is very important that you learn these rules.

4. Your institution has specific rules about the procedures to follow in developing a grant budget. These include allowable yearly salary increases, fringe benefit rates, allowable in-kind contributions, and the F&A cost-recovery rate. Knowing these rules prior to developing a grant application will save you considerable time in developing a budget.

5. In computing your budget, be as realistic as possible. Your budget should reflect your best estimate of the costs associated with each project activity. Do not over-estimate your budget and ask for too much. At the same time, do not underestimate the amount you will need to conduct your project.

6. Budgets usually contain three components: direct costs, F&A costs and institutional commitments. Categories in each of these components must be justified in a separate section of the budget.

Chapter 7

Technical Considerations

- Elements of a Concept Paper
- Needs Assessments and Pilot Efforts
- Obtaining Contractual Arrangements and Letters of Support

Knowledge of the technical aspects of writing a proposal can improve the competitiveness of your submission and save you valuable time in the proposal writing process. These include writing a concept paper, obtaining supporting documentation by conducting needs assessments or pilot studies, and attending to other administrative matters. In this chapter, we examine some of the common practices in grant writing that are learned through experience.

7.1 ELEMENTS OF A CONCEPT PAPER

Developing a concept paper before writing a full proposal is a strategy that many individuals find useful. A concept paper is similar to an extended abstract or an executive summary in that it outlines the major elements of the project you are developing. It is a brief document, comparable to a mini-proposal, containing many of the important elements of a full proposal. The concept paper is a very flexible tool that can help guide your proposal writing. It can be shared with multiple funding agencies, and allows you to receive feedback from a variety of sources. The key to a well-written concept paper is that it provides important information without burdening the reader with every detail that needs to be included in a full proposal. The Agency for Healthcare Research and Quality (AHRQ) recommends the length of a concept paper be six to 10 double-spaced pages, while other agencies recommend two to five double-spaced pages. In either case, the concept paper usually contains five basic sections as shown in Table 7-1. As you can see, these sections parallel many of the sections in a full proposal.

TABLE 7-1   Elements of a Concept Paper

1. Statement of Problem and Rationale
2. Research Question or Objectives
3. Methodology
4. Estimated Budget Requirements (not essential)
5. Key Personnel

The first section of a concept paper contains an introductory paragraph that describes the problem you plan to address and explains its importance or significance. Only a brief reference list of key citations should be included. This section is followed by a brief explanation of the specific aims or the short- and long-term objectives of the project. Then, describe the methodology you plan to use to attain the objectives. In a research project you would include a description of the study design, sampling procedures, sample size, data collection techniques, and analysis procedures. In an educational project, you would describe the steps you plan to take to conduct the project. You may then wish to include an estimated budget for the project with a brief justification of overall project costs. Although most agencies may not be interested in detailed budget information at this stage, providing an overall cost-estimate is helpful in evaluating whether your plan is feasible and consistent with the agency's funding levels. Finally, you will need to briefly identify the key participants in the project and their respective areas of expertise.

It may initially appear that writing a concept paper is unnecessary or a waste of time since its elements reflect the basic components of a grant application. However, taking the time to write such a paper has certain benefits, especially for a new investigator. Five major uses of for a concept paper are summarized in Table 7-2.

TABLE 7-2   Uses for a Concept Paper

- To aid discussion with federal project officer
- To submit to a foundation to determine interest
- To share with colleagues to obtain feedback
- To advance efforts of the grant writing team
- To assist in writing grant proposals as a working draft

First, some federal agencies may require a written statement regarding your intentions prior to submitting a full grant application. They may ask for either a "letter of intent," which is simply a letter stating that you intend to submit an application to the competition, or a more developed set of ideas in the form of a concept paper. If this is not required, it is still advantageous to send a concept paper to a program officer a few months in advance of the deadline for a particular competition. Program officers in most federal agencies will read and comment on your project if they receive a concept paper at least one month prior to the due date of a competition. However, be sure to call the agency first to determine their policy on reading and commenting on proposal ideas. Furthermore, if you plan to meet with a program officer, sending a concept paper via e-mail prior to your meeting will allow the program officer to review your ideas ahead of time so that you can both use your meeting time more effectively.

Second, the concept paper can be sent to program officers at foundations or to corporate leaders. Sending a concept paper with an introductory letter is often the preferred approach at many foundations. You may also send the paper to more than one foundation or corporation simultaneously, which will save you time in determining where there may be interest in your idea.

Third, the concept paper offers an easy way to obtain feedback from your colleagues. Since it is a brief document, it is not too time consuming for them to read. It enables you to obtain meaningful advice and suggestions without placing a burden on those who read it.

Fourth, the concept paper is an effective way to refine the thoughts of a team responsible for a grant submission. The paper represents an overview of the project. As such, it causes the group to focus on the feasibility of the grant idea and may help identify gaps that need to be addressed. It also helps the group formulate the next steps in developing the grant application.

Fifth, since the concept paper contains the basic elements of the grant application, it serves as the first working draft of the proposal. It can also be shared with individuals from whom you solicit letters of support for the application. Finally, aspects of the concept paper can be used to develop a submission to the institutional review board if human subjects are involved.

7.2 NEEDS ASSESSMENTS AND PILOT EFFORTS

In chapter 5, we emphasized the importance of demonstrating the significance of your idea and your expertise in the field of inquiry. An important way of demonstrating both points is conducting a pilot study and presenting your findings in a section of the proposal designated as either "Background and Significance," "Preliminary," or "Pilot Efforts."

The submission of an application for a demonstration, training, or education project usually requires that its significance be adequately demonstrated by a needs assessment. A needs assessment is a systematic approach for defining, analyzing, and evaluating a problem so that an intervention or an education program can be developed to target that need. A needs assessment provides data that define the nature and scope of the problem, identify the target population and ensure that a project is relevant.

For example, let's say you are proposing a continuing education program to advance the ability of practicing health professionals, such as occupational therapists and physical therapists, to provide family-centered care in early intervention programs in your region. To substantiate the need for such a program and its potential for improving services, it would be important to systematically survey the major early intervention programs in your region. Such an assessment might include the following:

a. the number of health professionals in the region who are working in early intervention programs

b. the number of health professionals in the region who are working in family centered care

c. the number of families currently receiving these services

   d. the number of families on waiting lists for these services

   e. the education level of practicing health professionals

   f. the level of knowledge in family-centered approaches to care

   g. family satisfaction with services they have received

   h. family perceptions of unmet needs

   i. willingness of practitioners to participate in a continuing education program on family centered care

   j. the number and type of educational opportunities in the region that are similar to the program you are proposing

The data obtained from this effort may provide evidence of personnel shortages, the lack of knowledge of family-centered care strategies by practitioners in the current system, and the need for continuing education programs. This evidence is critical to substantiate the need for a proposed continuing education program.

There are a range of methodological strategies that can be used to conduct a needs assessment. As in other types of research, the selection of a particular methodological approach for a needs assessment must fit the specific purpose, nature of the target population and the resources of the investigator. Table 7-3 describes a few of the methodological approaches that are commonly used to conduct a needs assessment.

Let's say you want to conduct an assessment of the need for an early intervention training program but you only have a relatively brief period of time, and you are limited in financial resources and personnel who are available to assist in the data collection effort. In this case, either a telephone interview or a mail survey of administrators of early intervention programs could be used to obtain the necessary data quickly. If time and personnel are not a barrier, however, then other methodologies might be considered. For example, a comprehensive survey of therapists, administrators, and family members can be conducted. This approach can be complemented by systematic observation of selected treatment sessions to evaluate the extent to which family-centered principles are integrated in practice. Another approach might involve conducting in-depth interviews with families to document their perceptions of the care they receive.

TABLE 7-3   Methodological Approaches Used in Needs Assessments

Method	Description
Delphi	Mail surveys to reach consensus about an issue from experts. Each expert indicates importance of items along a Likert-type scale through a number of iterations.
Focus Groups	Six to 15 individuals with similar backgrounds or experience are brought together to identify or discuss issues in a group. Types of focus groups include key informants, brainstorming, nominal group, and the use of either structured or semi-structured questions.
Interviews	Personal, face-to-face interviews using either structured, standardized questions or open-ended qualitative probes.
Mail Survey	Questionnaires sent by mail to a target population.
Telephone Surveys	Telephone interviews with a target population.
Document Reviews	Systematic review of literature, medical records, or other documents.
Direct Observation	Systematic observations of settings and behaviors.

If you plan to submit a proposal for a research study the inclusion of data collected from one or more pilot studies is very important. There are four major reasons for conducting a pilot study prior to the submission of a research grant application. As shown in Table 7-4, Pilot data can be used to demonstrate the potential significance of the project, enable the investigator to demonstrate his or her knowledge about the field of inquiry, test aspects of a research protocol, and obtain information about the target population.

TABLE 7-4   Reasons for Conducting a Pilot Study

---

1. To demonstrate the investigator's ability to conduct the proposed research and his or her familiarity with area
2. To pre-test the research design or other aspects of the methodology
3. To provide baseline data or preliminary information to justify the proposed effort and its significance
4. To increase the investigator's knowledge regarding the area of investigation

---

Beginning investigators may feel frustrated about the need to obtain pilot data since such efforts often require some level of funding or expenditure of effort. However, it is very important for beginning investigators to obtain preliminary data and develop a track record. Support for small research projects can be obtained from intramural competitions or department or institutional operating budgets. Investigators with a track record and who have received prior funding for a research study, are able to use the findings from these previous efforts as a basis for proposing a related research project. Obtaining pilot data does not have to be a costly activity. Collaborating with other researchers to conduct a mail or telephone survey, selected observations, focus groups, or in-depth interviews are cost-effective strategies that allow you to examine a clearly defined research question or test one aspect of the research protocol.

In presenting preliminary findings, it is important to indicate the way in which the pilot data supports the need for the study that is being proposed. Box 7-1 provides an excerpt from a grant application that illustrates how to report pilot findings.

7.3 OBTAINING CONTRACTUAL ARRANGEMENTS AND LETTERS OF SUPPORT

In addition to the narrative portion of the grant, there are other supplementary materials that need to be included in a proposal. For example, if you plan to have a formal work arrangement with another institution, you will need to sign a legal agreement in the form of a contract with that institution that clearly describes the working arrangement if the project is funded. In the application, you will need to include a letter of intent signed by an official of that institution. If your project requires a less formal arrangement or if there are individuals or groups whose participation or endorsement would be required or helpful, then letters of support should be included with your proposal.

BOX 7-1

PRELIMINARY STUDIES

The proposed research builds upon and significantly expands the previous research efforts of the investigators. Three studies in particular support the direction of the proposed effort and indicate its potential value.

Study #1 Dementia Management Study

The first study involved a two-group randomized design by which 220 caregivers of individuals with dementia were assigned to either a treatment or control group. Preliminary findings from 110 caregivers who completed the intervention indicate that an average of three caregiving problems were addressed. A total of 488 environmental strategies were suggested by the occupational therapist (OT) during the course of the five home visit interventions. OTs observed that caregivers used on average 83% or 406 of these strategies by the end of the intervention.

These preliminary findings suggest that caregivers can learn and adapt environmental strategies to fit their care situation and respond favorably to a home intervention that addresses individualized need. The intervention proposed in this application uses the environmental strategies that were developed in this study but tests their effectiveness with caregivers of individuals with stroke.

Contracts are usually handled by your institution. Most institutions require that you use standard forms that have been approved by institutional attorneys. If you are at a university, inquire at your office of research administration for these forms. Most university offices of research administration will complete these forms for you. If you are at another type of institution or agency, ask your director about the correct procedure. Be sure to specify in the contract all agreements that you have made with the other institution. These include the amount of money that will be paid, the payment schedule, the specific tasks that each party needs to complete in return for the money, and the time frame for completion of each task. Most institutions will require the legal department or head administrator to review and countersign the contract.

Letters of support must also be included in an application although they are less formal documents with fewer legal implications. A letter of support from a consultant assures the review panel that you do have the necessary support to carry out the project. For example, let's say you are submitting a proposal that involves working with persons who are homeless. Letters of support from administrators of homeless shelters, key personnel in city government who oversee programs for the homeless, and community leaders would be essential. In these letters you want to assure the funding agency that you have access to key resources, such as homeless shelters of study participants, or the endorsement of individuals or agencies knowledgeable about your project and important for its success. These letters are usually requested personally by a member of the project team. The concept paper, abstract, or first page of the specific aims can be sent to individuals so they have the information they need to write the letter and know what they are agreeing to participate in.

Both contracts and letters of support can be obtained early in the proposal process. One member of the team can be responsible for acquiring these, while other sections of the proposal, are being written. These letters and contracts are placed in an appendix of the final proposal, unless otherwise specified in the application instructions. These letters are then referred to in the document. A letter of support is usually addressed to the project director or principal investigator, and should include a reference to the title of the project and the name of the intended funding agency, along with the endorsement of the project.

7.4 ADMINISTRATIVE MATTERS

There are other administrative matter you must pay careful attention to when submitting a grant. Advanced knowledge of these matters can save time when you write the proposal and, in some cases, improve your chances of being funded.

a. *Boilerplate material*—Proposal writing is a time consuming activity. Developing a competitive idea, writing the proposal, and carrying out all the other related tasks takes considerable time. One way of cutting down on time is to prepare in advance basic information that is required in most proposals. This information is called "boilerplate material," because it is standard information and required in most grant applications. Examples of this material include descriptions of your institution's qualifications and resources, and the biographical sketches of project personnel. Such materials can be prepared in advance and then updated when necessary.

The section on institutional qualifications usually includes a series of brief paragraphs that contain a general description of the organization and mission of your institution, agency, college, school, or department. It also includes a description of resources such as the library, computer facilities, laboratories, institutional or agency affiliations, and any other components that make your organization special or demonstrate that the support you need for the success of the project is available. Most of this information can be found in your university catalog, annual report, or other public information developed by your agency. Consider developing two versions of this material, one relatively brief and another with more detail. Either version can then be modified and used in a grant proposal depending upon the depth required by a funding agency. Having the basic framework completed for this section of a grant will save you considerable time and effort.

The description of the qualifications of potential project team members is another example of boilerplate material that can be prepared in advance. There are two forms this may take. The first is a narrative biographical sketch. Ask members of your department or agency to write two biographical sketches, one long and the other short. The long version need not be more than three paragraphs and should contain a summary of their major accomplishments in research, teaching, and service. The short version can be a one paragraph description of these accomplishments. The second form is a standard biographical sketch, usually two or three pages, depending on the agency. This document contains your name, title, education history and a list of your publications, presentations, honors, and awards. NIH and other federal agencies require this form and the directions are included in the application instructions. As with the institutional qualifications, you will have to modify this sketch for each proposal to match the most appropriate skills of your team members to fit a particular project. However, advance preparation of the basic content will facilitate your grant writing effort.

b. *Typing the proposal*—When you write your proposal, make it pleasing to the eye and easy to read. If you have a page limitation, which most proposals do, avoid cramming extra information into the narrative by expanding your margins or using a smaller typeface. Most applications now require one inch margins and twelve point typeface. In addition, whatever advantage you may think you gain by the inclusion of extra information may be lost because of the fatigue and eyestrain experienced by the reviewers while reading your proposal. An attractive, organized, professional looking proposal enables a review panel to efficiently evaluate its content. Since most proposal writers have access to personal computers and laser jet printers that allow great flexibility in formatting and typeface, there is no excuse for submitting a sloppy proposal. Make sure that the printing is clear and crisp, the tables and graphs attractive and easy to read, and the punctuation, spacing, and headings logically consistent. Your proposal should be inviting to read. However, this does not imply that you should use colored graphs or fancy script. Colored graphs, when duplicated, will be black and white. Fancy script may hurt a reviewer's eyes after the first page. Do not right justify your narrative.

Right justification leaves too much white space and is more time consuming to read. So do not waste the reviewers' time and energy.

c. *Duplicating materials*—Most agencies require that you submit the original proposal and anywhere from two to eight copies. These copies must be complete and include all appendices and attachments. Sometimes agencies need more copies than are required by law, and it is helpful if you provide extra copies. Contact the program officer to inquire how many copies the agency would prefer you send. Agencies are on tight budgets and by sending extra copies, you will have saved your program officer or one of the secretaries valuable time and money. Duplicating an application is more time consuming than you may think. Consider completing the appendices several days to a week prior to the due date. This will allow you to duplicate these materials and eliminate the last minute rush and the stress that may be experienced.

d. *Requesting a special review*—If you believe that the nature of your proposal requires specific technical expertise, you can request that an individual with this specific expertise read your proposal as part of the review panel. This request can be made in a cover letter and the program officer will make a decision regarding the appropriateness of your request.

Some federal agencies will allow you to request that an additional agency, other than the one to which it is submitted, review your proposal. In other words, if you submit a proposal related to aging to the Agency for Healthcare Quality and Research, you could also request that the National Institute on Aging review the same proposal and serve as a second potential source for its funding. In the NIH, these requests should be made in your cover letter and then a Referral Officer will make such assignments.

e. *Mailing/delivering the proposal*—Once you have finished your proposal, it needs to be delivered to the agency on or before the published due date. The due date is specified in the general or supplemental instructions along with

the name and address of the office to which the proposal should be delivered and the number of copies to include. In the Department of Education, proposals must be post-marked on or before the due date. Some agencies in the Public Health Service, such as the Bureau of Health Professions, also follow this procedure. Other agencies, such as the National Institutes of Health, require that the proposals arrive in the Division of Research Grants on or before the due date.

Extensions on deadlines are never given. Therefore, pay close attention to the due date and determine the best method of delivery. If, in writing the proposal, you see that you will need up to the last minute possible for its completion, you may want to consider sending your proposal by a next day mail delivery service. Make sure that you obtain a receipt from the post office or courier that clearly shows the date and time of mailing. If your proposal is lost, this receipt is proof that it was mailed on time, and it will be accepted by the federal government and most foundations. You may also deliver your proposal personally. Investigators in institutions that are close to Washington, D.C., or the agency address often hand deliver their application. However, as long as the application arrives on time, there is no advantage to one or the other method of delivery.

f. *If you find a mistake*—After submitting your application, you may discover that you inadvertently neglected to include a particular appendix or that in duplication, the ordering of the document was disturbed. These kinds of errors are considered "small" and most agencies will correct these problems upon notification. Call the program officer to indicate the problem and to determine the best course of action.

g. *Plan for a resubmission*—Few proposals are funded on the first submission. Therefore, plan on submitting your proposal more than once. In resubmitting, listen to the advice of your program officer and be responsive to the suggestions of the review panel. (We discuss resubmitting your proposal in more detail in chapter 11.)

SUMMARY

In this section, technical considerations of proposal writing have been discussed, as well as administrative matters involved in the submission process. Four important points have been discussed.

1. Writing a concept paper can facilitate proposal development.

2. Needs assessments and pilot studies are essential, especially in today's competitive environment.

3. Writing a grant proposal is a time consuming activity. It is, therefore, important to plan a grant writing schedule in which you build contingencies. Among the often overlooked administrative details are such things as getting institutional approvals, duplicating an adequate number of copies, and delivering the proposal on time.

4. Developing boilerplate material is a valuable time saver. Boilerplate material includes descriptive narrative of institutional resources and qualifications of key personnel which can be kept on file and used for most grant proposals.

Chapter 8

Strategies for Effective Writing

- Organizing for the Writing Task
- Problems With Writing
- The Grant Writing Team

Well-written proposals, those that are clear, focused, and precise, have a greater chance of receiving a favorable review than those that are disorganized, unclear, and filled with typographical errors. Fortunately or unfortunately, the way you present your ideas sends a message to a review panel. Effective writing and an eye-pleasing presentation shows reviewers that you are conscientious, your ideas are important, and they have been carefully developed. Writing that is imprecise and rambling, or a presentation that is too dense or difficult to follow, can make it hard for reviewers to understand your reasoning and raise doubts about your ideas and, implicitly, your ability to implement the project. In addition, significant ideas may be misunderstood or missed by reviewers due to a writing style that is imprecise.

Although a clear writing style will not overcome a poor idea, it will help you sell a good one. However, a poorly written or presented proposal has the potential to hurt the chances of having a competitive idea funded.

As you write your proposal, it is important to understand four points about writing of any kind:

- First, while many people like to have written, few like to write. Writing is hard work. The old adage that good reading is hard writing, is true. Writing, like any other skill, takes practice. Improvement in writing only comes about through continual writing, rewriting, and critique. The more you write, the more improvement you will see in the quality of your writing.

- Second, you must be prepared to write, rewrite, and rewrite. A well-written grant proposal has been rewritten many times.

- Third, writing is a very idiosyncratic process. Each person has a particular writing style and a preferred work method. You will find that your own style and personal approach to organizing your work will emerge as you become more experienced at writing.

- Fourth, writing takes time. There are no shortcuts. You have to make the time to write. Few people can squeeze writing into a few moments here and there. This is an important point to keep in mind, since proposals have hard and fast deadlines. Therefore, you should plan a working schedule that allows sufficient time to develop and refine your ideas in written form.

While writing is an idiosyncratic process, it is also a systematic one that requires careful attention to the organization and logical presentation of thoughts. The use of words that precisely describe your ideas is critical. A proposal tells a "story" about what you plan to accomplish and how. The major points and essential details of the story must be clearly and concisely communicated.

There are several strategies that can be used to improve the quality of your written proposal. These include organizing the task, avoiding common writing problems and developing a grant writing team to facilitate the process. Let's examine each strategy.

8.1 ORGANIZING FOR THE WRITING TASK

One strategy that can improve your proposal writing is to develop a systematic plan of organization to accomplish the task. Box 8-1 outlines one approach you may find effective.

BOX 8-1

ORGANIZING THE WRITING TASK

1. Set aside a block of uninterrupted time
2. Outline the major sections of the proposal
3. Write an initial draft without worrying about grammar or style
4. Plan to write more than one draft
5. Critically evaluate your draft
6. Ask a colleague or consultant to critically evaluate the next to last draft

First, set aside a block of uninterrupted time to write. While we each have different work rhythms and styles, many people find that concentrated periods of two to three hours can be very productive. Shorter periods may not be long enough for you to get into a "writing flow." Periods longer than three hours can be very fatiguing. Trying to write when you are overly tired can be an unproductive and frustrating experience.

Second, start writing by outlining the major sections of the proposal. These sections should be based on the specific organizing format provided by the funding agency in the application kit, with special attention given to the evaluation criteria that will be used by the review panel. Begin by writing the section with which you are most comfortable or which you believe will be the easiest to tackle. You do not have to write each section in sequence. Writing the section that you are most comfortable with provides an immediate feeling of accomplishment and helps build momentum for the writing of other sections that may be more difficult.

Third, in the first draft, you should not worry about grammar or style. The purpose of this draft is to capture as many ideas on paper as possible. You will have the opportunity to concentrate on the technical aspects of your writing in subsequent drafts. You should consider this draft to be "for your eyes only." By doing so you will not have to worry about someone reading it and thinking you are a poor writer.

Fourth, plan to write at least four to six drafts of each section. Do not expect your first drafts to be perfect. Good writing requires re-writing, re-writing, and more re-writing. You might consider adopting the 2-2-2 rule: two drafts for initial ideas, sequencing, and logic; two drafts for critical reading, idea revision, and initial editing; and two drafts for final editing, refinement, and integration.

Fifth, once you complete a satisfactory draft of a section, put it aside for a day or two. This will help you examine it from a new perspective. When you come back to it, you may discover glaring mistakes in the logic of your presentation, ideas that are not clearly presented, or gaps in the proposed design. One strategy is to read aloud a section of the proposal, or tape record the reading and then listen carefully to it. This will give you a sense of what it sounds like to an outside reader. Another strategy is to visualize a review panel that has convened to discuss your proposal. Try to envision what a reviewer would say, especially if he or she was not familiar with your area of inquiry. These approaches all allow you to gain distance from your work and examine it from a more objective and critical perspective.

Finally, while you can learn to be a critical evaluator of your own drafts, it is also beneficial to obtain the perspective of others. After you have reread and edited the draft of a particular section, or even the entire proposal, ask a colleague or pay a consultant to provide a critical, careful review. The person you choose should have some familiarity with your topic and be willing and able to honestly appraise your work. You can significantly improve your writing skills by taking note of the comments others make about what you have written. Most writers get too close to their work and are unable to identify gaps in logic, missing explanations, or even fatal flaws in a project design. Obtaining constructive criticism about one's work is a difficult but important part of scholarship and an excellent way to improve your writing ability. However, hearing this critical commentary is perhaps one of the most painful or difficult aspects of scholarship. Nevertheless, it is an important component of the process and promotes learning and intellectual growth. Do not become defensive when someone has evaluated your work as less than perfect. Instead, pay close attention to their reactions and comments. These reactions and comments may be a good indicator of how a review panel will receive your ideas.

8.2 PROBLEMS WITH WRITING

The second way to improve the quality of your proposal is to avoid problems that are commonly found in writing. A major problem many people have in writing is that they do not use language in a precise manner. Proposal writing is not a time to be fancy or experimental in language use and composition. A proposal requires a scientific, technical approach to writing in which the details of your project are clearly described. The proposal narrative should not be cluttered with non-essential material or extraneous words. Decide which details are the most important to include and incorporate them. Extraneous phrases and words make it difficult for a reviewer to understand your main points. Brevity, clarity, and organization are the keys to good proposal writing.

Listed in Box 8-2 are nine specific rules to facilitate clear writing.

BOX 8-2

SOME RULES FOR CLEAR WRITING
1. Stay away from jargon
2. Avoid words that are "trendy"
3. Do not use abbreviations such as "etc."
4. Avoid colloquialisms
5. Do not try to sound "intellectual" by using big words
6. Avoid redundant phrases
7. Keep over-used phrases to a minimum
8. Watch for unclear referents
9. Define core constructs/variables and relevant terms and use consistent wording throughout the proposal

1. *Stay away from jargon.* Using jargon is an imprecise approach to writing. Phrases like "meeting the needs of all patients" or "research that will address the health needs of the American people," have very little meaning. What specific needs are you going to meet?

2. *Avoid words that are "trendy."* There are many phrases that should only be used with caution in grant proposals. These include the following: "cutting edge," "state of the art," "vis-a-vis," "in-depth," "conceptual framework," "innovative." What does the following sentence really mean: "A state-of-the-art, cutting edge, innovative conceptual framework will be developed vis-a-vis this study." If you do use words such as "innovative" or "cutting edge," then you need to carefully and clearly explain how or in what way the program is innovative or on the cutting edge. For example, you could say "This program is innovative in that it brings together health professionals and academic faculty to work together to develop a curriculum for students." In this way, you clearly specify the aspect of the program that you consider to be innovative.

   Also, do not assume that the reviewer will know the common words used in your profession. If you do use the jargon of your field, be sure to carefully define and explain the terms. For example, researchers in one profession have used the phrase "calibrating raters" when they refer to ensuring that two different raters are consistent in their evaluation of a particular condition. This process is the same as assessing inter-rater reliability, which is a term commonly used among social scientists. Since calibration is usually used to refer to an instrument, a review panel could be confused about the use of this term if it is not adequately explained.

3. *Do not try to cut corners by using abbreviations* such as "etc." (e.g., women with dependent children, adolescents, teenagers, etc., commonly cited as "runaways . . . "). Using abbreviations is a lazy way of writing and reflects an inadequate development of your thoughts. In this example, are there others who would be classified as runaways? If so, the complete definition should be given. If not, the abbreviation, "etc." is unnecessary.

4. *Avoid colloquialisms.* You are writing a scientific proposal, so phrases such as, "The findings from these studies were great!" or "The researchers had a notion to study homelessness," are imprecise and inappropriate.

5. *Do not try to sound "intellectual."* It is not necessary to use a word with three syllables (utilize) when a one-syllable word (use) is adequate. Box 8-3 contains seven phrases that are commonly used but that can be restated to reflect an idea more accurately.

BOX 8-3

EXAMPLES OF EFFICIENT WRITING

Don't use	When you can use
an excessive amount of	too much
at a high level of productivity	highly productive
at a rapid rate	rapidly
due to the fact that	because
has the capability of	can
in view of the fact that	since
serves the function of being	is

6. *Avoid redundant phrases.* A point only needs to be made once. For example, phrases like "period of time," "green in color," "basic, fundamental essential," "audible to the ear," and "demographic statistical data" are examples of redundant phrases.

7. *Keep over-used phrases to a minimum.* Phrases such as the following tend to be over-used in proposals: "a thorough search of the literature," "an in-depth study," "a large body of information," "in the final analysis." Although the use of these phrases may be appropriate at times, they are often an indication of inadequate development of one's thoughts.

8. *Watch for unclear referents.* The use of unclear referents is a common problem that occurs when you begin a sentence with a pronoun that refers to someone or something

in the preceding sentence. An example of an unclear reference is shown in Box 8-4. In this example, it is unclear to whom the words "they" and "their" in the second sentence refer. Do these words refer to health professionals or the homeless that are discussed in the previous sentence?

BOX 8-4

EXAMPLE OF AN UNCLEAR REFERENT

The homeless are among the most disenfranchised and underserved who could greatly benefit from the services of health and human services professionals. *They* would contribute significantly to *their* health and well-being.

8.3 THE GRANT WRITING TEAM

Another strategy to enhance the effectiveness of your proposal writing is to organize a grant writing team. As we have said before, writing a proposal can be time consuming and arduous. There are myriad details involved in putting together a grant application. Often, it is helpful to share the writing and other responsibilities with members of a team, each of whom can be assigned a specific writing responsibility. A grant writing team enables individuals to "share the pain of writing" and carry out other activities that will expedite the completion of a proposal. An added advantage of this approach is that it assigns writing responsibilities based on each member's area of knowledge and skills. For example, if one member of your team has an interest and expertise in curriculum development, he or she can be assigned to write the initial draft of the curriculum objectives. In a research proposal, the statistician on your team can write the statistical analysis section. In an interdisciplinary team, a literature review from each discipline can be written by the representative of that discipline.

With this team approach, members of the team can also be assigned roles other than writing. For example, if an individual has contact with clinical affiliates or government agencies, then this person can be assigned to collect letters of support from these organizations.

Organizing a grant writing team that fills the following 10 roles can be an effective strategy. These roles represent the most common tasks required to develop most grant proposals. Each member of the team may be assigned more than one role, so it is not necessary to create a 10-member team. Focusing on these roles will help you organize your time and schedule important activities that need to be accomplished. Two to four members will usually suffice to complete a proposal efficiently.

BOX 8-5

ROLES ON A GRANT WRITING TEAM

1. Proposal coordinator/director
2. Agency contact person
3. Draft writers
4. Editor
5. Final draft writer
6. Budget coordinator
7. Coordinator of references
8. Coordinator of letters of support
9. Graphics coordinator
10. Typist and proofreader

---

1. Proposal coordinator/director—The person in this role assumes responsibility for the overall coordination of the proposal writing effort. He or she organizes the project and assures that members complete their assigned tasks in a timely manner. This individual often is the person who will be the principal investigator or director of the project when it is funded.

2. Agency contact person—The agency contact person serves as liaison with the funding agency. While writing the proposal, you may need to contact the program officer to

obtain feedback on the project idea, clarify the requirements of the competition, or inquire about technical matters as they emerge in the process of developing the
application. Communication with the program officer
should be handled by one member of the team. Usually
this role is assigned to the proposal coordinator or principal investigator. However, it could also be assumed by
another member of the team who is familiar with the
agency or who has had previous contact with the program
officer. A program officer can then associate the proposal
with one person rather than several, and will not have to
repeat advice or suggestions.

3. Draft writer—The first and second drafts of the proposal
   are usually the most difficult to write. At this stage, members of the team should be assigned to different sections
   of the proposal and assume responsibility for writing an
   initial draft of each. For example, a member of the team
   with expertise in curriculum development should be
   assigned the responsibility of writing the first draft of the
   program goals and objectives. Other members might be
   more knowledgeable about research methodology or
   experienced at conducting literature reviews. Individuals
   should write the first draft of those sections for which they
   have the most knowledge or skill.

4. Editor—Either a member of the team or an outside expert
   can serve as an editor. An editor reads for accuracy of content and comprehensiveness, as well as for grammar and
   punctuation, style, and format. He or she assumes the role
   of critic and has the responsibility of identifying gaps in conceptual development and/or unclear writing. Usually, it is
   best to edit for conceptual development and completeness
   in earlier drafts and grammar and punctuation in later drafts.

5. Final draft writer—Since writers have different styles, one
   person must take responsibility for assuring continuity in
   writing, particularly in the use of terminology and language. This person should write the later drafts after all
   decisions about content have been made by the team. The
   editor or proposal coordinator often serves in this role.

6. Budget coordinator—One person, usually the principal
   investigator, should be in charge of developing the budget
   and obtaining the necessary institutional approvals if your

institution does not have a designated individual assigned to this task. Once discussions have been held about the scope of the budget, it can be developed independently of the narrative sections of the proposal. Therefore, it can be submitted and approved by the appropriate institutional officials at any time and does not have to wait until the narrative is completed.

7. Coordinator of references—One person can be assigned the responsibility of assuring that references are properly cited and presented in a consistent format. This is a time-consuming but important job and one that can begin as soon as an initial draft is completed. There are various computer software programs, such as Reference Manager, that are available to assist you in the organization of citations. These programs are wise investments since they can help you complete this task in an efficient way.

8. Coordinator of letters of support—Obtaining letters of support from individuals or agencies who will be involved in your project is another important detail that can be time-consuming. This is a task that can be tackled early in the grant writing process. You should obtain letters from your congressmen, individuals in your organization assuring institutional commitment, consultants, or organizations that will be participating in your program. One member of the team should be assigned the responsibility for contacting these individuals and collecting their letters.

9. Graphics coordinator—Using tables and graphs can effectively summarize your points and concisely organize important information. Grant charts that present a timeline of the project activities and the involvement of key personnel, and figures that display the research or curriculum design are just some of the graphics you may want to include in your proposal. If you do not have a graphics software program, it is worth the price to have these materials developed by experts. Drafts of this material can be developed during the early stages of proposal writing and then revised, if necessary. One member of the grant writing team can assume responsibility for developing the initial drafts of these materials and coordinating the effort to have the materials developed.

10. Typist and proofreader—This is a very important role in the development of a competitive proposal. Someone who can format the final draft and proofread the proposal for consistency in presentation is an invaluable asset to a grant writing team. This can be a time consuming task so allow enough time for proofreading, formatting, and printing the final version on the correct forms.

A grant writing team can be an effective way of organizing the submission of a proposal, particularly for those that require the participation of different disciplines or individuals with diverse areas of expertise. Nevertheless, there are two points to keep in mind if you use this approach. First, some team members who participate in writing drafts may be sensitive to criticism about their writing style and may feel insulted when their draft is reworked. Because of the potential problems that may occur, members of the team need to be aware that the grant writing process involves constant revision and modification, and that the sections they contribute will be revised a number of times.

Second, it is essential that the members of the grant writing team complete their assigned tasks in a timely and efficient manner. The due date for a grant submission is not negotiable and the deadlines for initial drafts and other assignments must be treated seriously.

SUMMARY

Well written proposals are those in which ideas are presented clearly, concisely, and logically. Such proposals have a greater chance of receiving a favorable review than those that are disorganized, unclear, and filled with typographical errors. This chapter presents three strategies to improve the quality of your written proposal.

1. Develop a systematic approach to writing. We discussed six organizational strategies to help in this book.

2. Avoid common mistakes in writing. Nine rules for improving your writing were presented.

3. Consider developing a team to work together in submitting a grant application. We outlined 10 roles that individuals can assume on a grant writing team.

Part IV

Models for Proposal Development

Compared to other disciplines, the health and human service professions are in an initial stage of development in competing for external sources of support. This is, in part, due to a lack of experience in grantsmanship, the lack of available federal funds that are earmarked specifically for health professionals, and the complexity of the professional lives of health and human service academics and practitioners. Whereas grantsmanship is often the primary work of social and behavioral scientists, health and human service professionals must delicately balance multiple roles. These roles include training students to become practitioners, providing direct services or administering these services, and participating in the scientific advancement of practice. Each of these roles are time consuming, compete for a professional's focused energies, and require a different set of skills and expertise. Thus, the multiple roles of health and human service professionals pose a special challenge and necessitate a different, organized approach to grantsmanship than that traditionally used in the social and medical sciences.

For this reason, we believe the next two chapters are very important and provide meaningful strategies to enable professionals in both academic and practice settings to participate in the process of obtaining external funds. Chapter 9 introduces four different organizational structures for developing proposal ideas and submitting grant applications. These structures are conceptualized along a continuum from individual to collaborative team efforts. The benefits of each, and the particular circumstances under which they are most effective, are also discussed. Chapter 10 describes in more depth a collaborative, team approach to project development. A collaborative project structure is particularly timely in that it is embedded in many funding priorities and facilitates the development of complex, multi-faceted educational and research programs in the health and human services. We present a model to guide the collaborative process that is based on the framework of social exchange theory and the team building literature. The model offers a basis for bridging research and practice settings or enabling individuals from different disciplines or distinct areas of expertise to effectively work together. Knowledge of the range of organizational approaches and the collaborative process enables individuals, departments, and institutions to develop the necessary infrastructure to support grantsmanship.

Chapter 9

Four Project Structures

- Individual Project Model
- Consultative Project Model
- Cooperative Model
- Collaborative Model
- Choosing an Appropriate Project Structure

Now that you are familiar with various strategies for identifying a funding source and writing a grant proposal, it is important to consider other key aspects of project development and implementation. The successful development and implementation of a research or educational project not only requires knowledge of grantsmanship, but also the ability to organize and manage a project staff with distinct areas of expertise. Each research or training project differs in the number and complexity of its activities, the type and amount of coordination required, and the skills that must be possessed by the project staff. To be successful, the principal investigator or project director must structure the project in such a way as to maximize efficiency in striving for successful project implementation.

There are basically four distinct models by which to organize research or training grants. We refer to these as individual, consultative, cooperative, and collaborative. Each approach has a set of defining characteristics, is useful under different circumstances, and has unique advantages and disadvantages. Understanding different approaches to project development and management will help you implement an organizational approach that best fits your preferred style, the nature of the project, and your institutional environment. Although it is possible to use one approach in project development and then another once the project is funded, usually one organizational model will be used at both the grant writing and project implementation stages.

The four models of project organization can be conceptualized along a continuum based on the degree to which individuals are involved in the project. On one end of the continuum is an individualized work effort in which there is minimal involvement of others. On the other end is a collaborative structure that is team oriented and requires the greatest organizational effort and level of involvement of participants. Each of these project structures can be defined by the extent to which 14 basic characteristics are present. These characteristics are summarized in Table 9.1. Let's examine each model.

9.1 INDIVIDUAL MODEL

An individual model reflects the "traditional" academic approach. In this model, a single investigator works independently to develop and carry out a research or, in some cases, an educational project. An individual model contains only one of the defining characteristics found in Table 9.1, that of a clear statement of goals, expectations, and procedures. Although this characteristic is a basic requirement of any project, it serves different purposes within each organizational model. In the individual model, a clear statement of goals, expectations, and procedures helps an investigator remain focused and task-oriented in carrying out the activities of the project. An individual approach is effective and appropriate in at least four situations:

1. Small pilot grant efforts, especially those under $50,000

2. The individual is an experienced investigator with a well-developed research agenda and is an expert in all facets of the project

3. Competitions in which the purpose is to advance an individual's career (fellowships, special training opportunities, postdoctorates, mentored or internship awards)

4. Discrete pieces of research, such as the structure of protein molecules in a laboratory, an investigation of the outcomes of a particular educational strategy in the classroom, or the development or advancement of a particular theoretical framework

An individual work model is less viable for large projects that necessitate the involvement of diverse areas of expertise and experience or require the participation of more than one organization. In fact, it is becoming increasingly more difficult for one person to have the knowledge and expertise in every facet of a project and the time to keep abreast of the literature in fields that may be relevant to the core project idea. The traditional picture of the lone researcher working in his or her laboratory, developing a brilliant research project is not an effective or realistic one for the beginning investigator. Also, with the exception of those situations described above, working alone can be an isolating experience that lacks intellectual stimulation.

TABLE 9.1   Fourteen Defining Characteristics of Project Structures

Defining Characteristics	Individual	Consultative	Cooperative	Collaborative
Clear statement of goals, expectations, procedures	xxx	xxx	xxx	xxx
Differentiation of roles		x	xx	xxx
Open communication		x	x	xxx
Open, honest negotiation		xx	xx	xxx
Mutual goals			xx	xxx
Climate of trust		x	xx	xxx
Cooperation		x	xx	xxx
Shared decision making			x	xx
Conflict resolution			xx	xxx
Equality of participation				xx
Group cohesion				xx
Decision by consensus				xx
Shared leadership				xx
Shared responsibility for participation				xx

Note: x's indicate the presence of a characteristic and the level of its intensity with more x's indicating greater intensity.

9.2 CONSULTATIVE MODEL

A consultative model is an extension of the individual approach. An investigator using this model develops a project idea and then requests assistance from experts or consultants who can contribute specific expertise or skills. Consultants may be hired to write a discrete section of a proposal or perform a particular activity for a project that is funded. They do not "own" the project idea, but contribute their expertise to enhance one particular aspect of it. The involvement of a consultant is usually viewed favorably by a review panel because the additional expertise increases the likelihood of the successful completion of the project.

Let's say you want to conduct a cost-effectiveness analysis in a study that tests a health service program. However, you do not have expertise in cost effectiveness analysis. You would need to find an expert in this area to serve as a consultant. In order to work effectively with you, the consultant would need to become familiar with the general purposes and objectives of your program in order to determine the variables that are most appropriate to include in a cost analysis. However, he or she might have little interest in or need to understand your theoretical framework or how the program contributes to the scholarly base in your field.

A consultative model of organization has six defining characteristics: a clear statement of project goals, expectations, and procedures; differentiation of roles; open communication; open and honest negotiation; a climate of trust; and cooperation. The need for a clear statement of goals and expectations is important to help guide the overall project and identify the specific responsibilities of your consultant. Therefore, your responsibility to the consultant is to explain the project in a clear and concise fashion and describe specifically your expectations for his or her work effort.

A second characteristic, role differentiation, can be defined as a set of procedures and roles assigned to individuals to guide their behavior in carrying out specific tasks of the project (we discuss this concept in more detail in chapter 10). In organizing a project using a consultative model, the specific responsibilities of the consultant must be clearly communicated so that the work can be performed effectively.

Although it is important to identify a consultant with whom you can work productively, it is also important for you to solidify the working relationship by communicating openly and negotiating fairly. A relationship that is characterized by open communication and involves honest negotiation about the nature and scope of work will help you arrive at a mutually satisfying agreement and a working climate that is productive. The relationship must also involve a level of trust and cooperation so that tasks are performed in a timely and effective manner and fit your expectations as to what must be accomplished. The agreement with the consultant should be outlined in a legally binding contract that indicates the scope of the work, the time line for its completion, and the method of payment. This document is often referred to as a professional consulting agreement. Most consultative agreements will indicate that the consultant does not have intellectual ownership of any part of the study or the product that they provide as part of the scope of work, and that they are not permitted to use or publish the materials without obtaining prior written permission from the principal investigator. Most universities or major institutions will have standard agreement forms that have been reviewed and approved by their legal department.

A consultative model is most effective for projects in which you have adequate knowledge and skill to carry out the major activities, but there is a need for technical expertise in a specified and well-defined area. This model is appropriate for individuals in social service agencies or health care facilities who may have knowledge about the major topic of a project but need assistance either in developing and implementing evaluation techniques, research design, or data analysis. Most large projects will require the use of one or more consultants.

9.3 COOPERATIVE MODEL

A cooperative model is an extension of a consultative approach. There are two types of cooperative models. In one type, an investigator identifies an idea for a project and invites one or more individuals in the same or other disciplines at his or her institution to work on major aspects of it. The initiator of the project defines the scope of involvement of each member and directs the group's activities. A second form of this model involves a cooperative arrangement among two or more institutions. The initiating or lead institution takes overall responsibility for the conduct of the project and defines the involvement of the other institution(s) in the form of a legal contract. In both types, all parties need to establish a systematic approach to organizing the project and create a productive working relationship. Participants divide the project into discrete areas of responsibilities and tasks. Members of the group then meet periodically to report their progress in carrying out their responsibilities and to make decisions about the project. Although participants work closely together, they do so as individuals, each assuming responsibility for his or her particular area. The end product of this "working group" reflects each individual's unique contribution and is an additive approach to problem solving.

Occasionally, a funding agency will seek a cooperative agreement with a grantee. In this case, the sponsor typically announces a particular request for applications in which such an arrangement is specified prior to the grant submission. In such a cooperative agreement, the funding agency has a major role in decision-making as to the conduct of the funded science or educational program. This is an example of an organizational structure based on a cooperative model.

A cooperative model contains nine of the defining characteristics outlined in Table 9.1. As in each of the other organizational models, cooperative arrangements are based on a clear statement of goals, expectations, and procedures that defines the direction of the project and its management. In this model, role differentiation becomes even more important than in the other work models. The cooperating groups must have a clear understanding of work expectations and the specific tasks that each needs to accomplish. This working relationship requires cooperation, open communication, honest negotiation, and professional respect or trust if it is to be successful. The possibility of disagreement exists in any working relationship; therefore, participating parties must also develop an effective mechanism for making decisions and resolving conflict.

A cooperative model is effective in projects involving multiple and distinct tasks, a clear division of labor, and distinct work performed by each participating institution or group separately. A cooperative arrangement can strengthen a project because it brings together individuals with complementary strengths and resources from different disciplines or institutions to carry out the project. Funding agencies often encourage projects that are organized according to this model because it allows for meaningful contributions by many individuals or institutions that would otherwise not be available in an individual or consultative project structure. This is particularly the case for research projects that require the recruitment of a particular population, which may be difficult to achieve from one geographic region.

Box 9.1 provides an example of a project in which a cooperative model would be appropriate.

BOX 9-1

CASE EXAMPLE OF A COOPERATIVE MODEL

Dr. S., an associate professor in physical therapy, is interested in working with young children with disabilities. She has developed a set of protocols that have been tested and shown to be effective. Dr. S. wants to demonstrate the effectiveness of her protocols in the public school setting, but she does not have access to a sufficient number of schools nor the experience in developing training materials that are appropriate to that setting. Dr. S. decides to contact a colleague, Dr. T., who is a faculty member in a school of education in another region who has done extensive work with schoolteachers. She discusses her ideas with Dr. T., who is interested in expanding her contacts in the schools and who agrees to cooperate on the project. Dr. S. submits a grant in which her institution is the applicant organization. She involves Dr. T. and her institution as part of a consortium relationship. That is, a sub-award will be established with Dr. T.'s institution that supports the work effort of Dr. T. and her team.

As you can see in the example above, Dr. S. has specific knowledge that is useful to teachers working with children who have disabilities. However, she lacks experience with teachers and, most importantly, the network by which to disseminate materials within school districts. Dr. T. has worked extensively with schoolteachers, is familiar with public school districts, and has developed teacher-training materials. Dr. S. and Dr. T. have complementary perspectives, skills, and resources. Each has access to different networks of experts, trainees, and bodies of literature and each can accomplish a discrete work effort that addresses each of their own goals, while contributing to the accomplishment of the overall project. Therefore, both benefit from a cooperative arrangement. As part of the subcontract to Dr. T.'s institution, direct and indirect costs are requested so that both institutions benefit from this arrangement.

9.4 COLLABORATIVE MODEL

A collaborative model builds on a cooperative approach and involves a more complex organizational structure. Whereas cooperative models are built around working groups in which each individual contributes to the completion of a task, a collaborative model relies on the development of a "team" to work on all aspects of the project, from planning to implementation. Teams are different from working groups. Working groups are based on a collection of individual actions in which performance is a function of what members do as individuals. The focus is on individual work products, and each participant is accountable for the final product. In a collaborative, team-based model, there is interdependent problem solving and task performance. Successful performance requires both individual and collective actions. Collective work products reflect the joint or integrated contributions of team members, and both the individual and the group are mutually accountable (Katzenbach & Smith, 1993). Teams may be composed of health and human service professionals from the same or different disciplines, faculty members and clinicians, researchers and consumers, or any combination of these individuals.

There are many definitions of collaboration. Katzenbach and Smith (1993, p. 112) define collaboration as "a small number of people with complementary skills who are committed to a common purpose, set of performance goals, and approach for which they hold themselves mutually accountable." This definition highlights the importance of teams having "complementary skills" and a commitment to a common purpose or mutual goal.

Whitney (1990, p. 11) provides another way of understanding collaboration. She suggests that "real collaboration involves at least two different sets of ideas, known goals to be reached by each collaborator, differing and complementary talents, and a good measure of individual passion to continually generate, combine, and separate activities in response to both individual and group goals." This definition emphasizes the importance of combining different ideas and the passion, energy, and commitment that is necessary to meet the challenges of the constantly changing dynamic of individuals interacting in groups.

We build on these definitions and view collaboration as "an indepth cooperative effort in which experts from the same or different disciplines are linked in such a way that they build on each other's strengths, backgrounds, and experiences and together develop an integrative approach to resolve a research or educational problem." Thus, "problem formulation and solutions reflect a perspective that is more than the sum of each participant's contribution." (Gitlin, Lyons, & Kolodner, 1994, p. 16).

Our definition emphasizes the importance of integrating ideas. That is, in a collaborative effort, experts work together in such a way as to build on each other's strengths, backgrounds, and experiences, so that an integrative approach to a research, education, or training problem is achieved. Using this approach, individuals with mutual interests but perhaps different areas of expertise meet to explore potential project and proposal ideas. These individuals work closely to jointly define and develop the project idea and a plan for its implementation. Ideas for a project emerge from the interaction and exchange of individuals. Each person on a collaborative team combines his or her skills with those of other team members in such a way that problems may be redefined and solutions found that reflect multiple levels of expertise and knowledge. The final project idea and plan for implementation represents the integration of multiple perspectives and is thus the product of the group interaction. Solutions identified through this approach are much different than those that would be identified by using an additive approach to problem solving—that is, the whole is greater than the sum of its parts.

A collaborative work model contains the nine defining characteristics of a cooperative model, but to a greater degree of intensity. For example, although open and honest negotiation may be present in consultative and cooperative models, this characteristic is critical for the effective development of a collaborative team. Group deliberations must be honest and open for a team to learn about and integrate each member's opinion and expertise. This is not a necessary requirement for the success of a cooperative or consultative model.

A collaborative approach is also characterized by five unique characteristics: equality of participation, decision making through consensus, shared leadership, shared responsibility for participation, and group cohesion. Equality of participation is particularly important because program ideas emerge from the blending or integration of the viewpoints of all team members. All members of the team bring critical expertise to the project and therefore are essential for its effective completion. Because of the importance of these skills, each member must be seen as an equal contributor to the team's deliberations. Teams that reinforce equality of participation will also seek to involve all members in decision making and recognize the value of reaching a consensus on major decisions. When members make contributions in their respective areas of expertise, they are assuming a leadership role. As individuals become more involved in decisions, they will also develop a responsibility for participation because their contributions to team decisions are seen as important to the group. These processes result in the emergence of a high level of group cohesion that, in turn, leads to an environment or climate of trust, in which conflicts can be openly addressed and members feel free to make important contributions to the grant-writing process.

The five major advantages to this organizational model are summarized in Table 9.2.

TABLE 9.2   Advantages of a Collaborative Model

1. Provides mentoring experience
2. Enables efficient use of limited resources
3. Provides a competitive advantage for certain funding programs
4. Facilitates interdisciplinary interaction
5. Enables multisite participation and development of more complex projects

First, a collaborative approach provides an important mentoring opportunity for individuals on the team who may be less experienced in grant writing and/or conducting funded projects. Through participation and inclusion as a collaborator, an inexperienced faculty member, clinician, or service provider gains invaluable firsthand knowledge and skills. Second, a collaborative approach overcomes limited resources, such as the lack of specialized knowledge and experience, which are major barriers to grant writing in the health and human service professions. Also, the rapid advancement of scientific knowledge makes it difficult for any one person to have all the information necessary to carry out a complex project. Third, an interdisciplinary approach can provide a competitive advantage since many funding agencies are now encouraging interdisciplinary approaches to projects. Fourth, the development of a team of collaborators promotes interdisciplinary sharing of knowledge as opposed to the multidisciplinary participation that exists in a cooperative or consultative arrangement. Interdisciplinary collaboration allows members of one discipline to learn about and come to respect the potential contributions of those in other disciplines. Finally, as in a cooperative arrangement, collaboration enables a team to develop more complex education and research projects that may involve the participation of different disciplines or multiple sites. Complex projects such as curriculum development, cost-benefit, or statistical analyses require more specialized skills that many investigators do not possess. As Katzenbach and Smith (1993) suggest, the real purpose of a collaborative team is to be "cutting edge," "revolutionizing," and "first!"

Nevertheless, it should be noted that a collaborative model still requires that one person be designated as the leader, most often the principal investigator of the grant project. The leader will ultimately be responsible for the integrity of the science or education program. A collaborative approach does not negate recognition of a hierarchical structure in which the principal investigator has the final decision-making authority.

Despite the potential benefits of a collaborative approach, there are several disadvantages. First, collaboration is time-consuming in that it involves organizing and integrating the contributions of many individuals. It requires a very strong leader (e.g., principal investigator or project director) who has the skills to develop and foster a team approach and who can strike an effective balance in independent decision-making and team involvement. Second, some individuals may not be able to participate in shared decision making or may not have a personality that lends itself to compromise and revision. Third, collaborative projects may cost more to implement, because they involve the coordination of more individuals and necessitate frequent meetings. Finally, many academic disciplines, including those in the health and human service fields, are primarily concerned with their own professional advancement. This unidisciplinary focus often discourages team-oriented approaches in research or education.

9.5 CHOOSING AN APPROPRIATE PROJECT STRUCTURE

The four work styles—individual, consultative, cooperative, and collaborative—offer diverse but also complementary approaches to developing a project idea and a grant application. One work style and organizational model is not necessarily superior or more effective than the other. The selection of an organization model depends on the nature of the idea, the complexity and size of a project, the experience of the individuals involved, and the resources available. One model does not necessarily exclude the other. For example, a consultative approach can be integrated into the other models. Also, occasionally a collaborative model for a complex project may require that certain activities be organized to reflect a more individualized working style.

One way to choose the most appropriate organizational structure is to consider how much involvement of others is necessary. This can be determined by asking yourself these questions:

- Do I have the necessary skills or knowledge to carry out my idea?
- Do I have the time to complete the tasks that will be required?
- Do I have the resources needed to complete the project?

If you are lacking a specific skill, area of knowledge, time, or resources, then you should consider involving others who are capable of filling these gaps. This informal needs assessment will suggest the size and composition of your project team and the model of project organization that may be most effective.

Unfortunately, a "do it alone" attitude continues to impose a significant barrier to the health and human service professions in their efforts to advance their professions through systematic inquiry. A narrow, discipline-specific approach shortchanges the professions in that problem formulation based solely in the academic environment frequently lacks relevance to daily clinical issues or results in program designs that are inappropriate for a practice setting. A unidisciplinary perspective also limits the potential growth of any one discipline in that it precludes the intellectual stimulation that results from interactions with others.

An individual-based approach to research and education also shortchanges clinicians or practitioners who usually do not have the resources, in terms of time and research knowledge, to engage in a research or education project. Finally, the approach also shortchanges consumers. Many agencies require that consumers be involved in the planning and implementation of programs developed by health and human service professionals. Consumers have a unique perspective and a different understanding of their own needs than do "outside experts." A productive approach for the health and human service professions is to consider a team approach that involves the equal participation of practitioners and academic faculty.

Team approaches can address many of the issues faced by health and human service professionals as they strive to improve their ability to acquire outside funding. These issues include lack of experience in grant writing, the scarcity of doctoral prepared investigators, and the lack of resources. A collaborative model has the potential to improve the skills of inexperienced faculty and practitioners and bridge the gap between the academic and clinical environments to advance research, service, and education in the health and human service fields. Although most faculty members are familiar with individual and consultative arrangements, cooperative and collaborative models may offer all professionals greater opportunities to improve their writing and project development skills.

Chapter 10

Understanding the Process of Collaboration

- Theoretical Framework for Understanding Collaboration
- Roles and Responsibilities of Team Members
- Five-Stage Model of Collaboration
- Evaluating Indicators of Collaboration
- Problems and Solutions

Multidisciplinary and collaborative teamwork has received significant attention in the health and human services literature in recent years. Numerous federal agencies and foundations have begun to emphasize a collaborative approach in program announcements and requests for applications (RFA). Collaborating and working with a team requires a working style that is distinct from what we described in the last chapter as "individual" or "consultative." One must develop a team orientation to problem-solving and an interdependent approach to accomplishing specific tasks. For those who are used to working alone, initially group participation will be unfamiliar and appear difficult and time consuming. To some it will seem painful. It is not surprising that collaboration has been defined by some as "an unnatural act between two or more unconsenting adults!"

Nevertheless, as we have discussed in chapter 9, for certain projects, a collaborative approach is an effective working model, and one that should be considered. Although it may at first appear to be a cumbersome approach, it is possible to learn how to work effectively on a team and benefit from group participation. An understanding of the process of collaboration will enable you to become a more competent participant and effective leader of such an effort.

In this chapter we discuss the development and dynamics of collaborative teams. We first present a brief discussion of a theoretical framework that provides a rationale for collaborative behavior. This framework uses two important concepts that facilitate the evolution and functioning of a collaborative group structure, role differentiation, and role releases. We then compare roles assumed on a traditional research project with ones that emerge in a collaborative team and discuss the responsibilities of a team leader. Based on this framework, we present a five-stage model of collaboration that explains the process by which collaborative groups emerge and teamwork is sustained. We also discuss ways to evaluate collaborative functioning, identify problems that might arise in teams and suggest ways these problems may be addressed.

10.1 TECHNICAL FRAMEWORK FOR UNDERSTANDING COLLABORATION

To understand the collaborative process, it is helpful to examine the ways individuals behave in groups and how groups, in turn, shape the exchanges that occur among their members. Social exchange theory and the literature on team building are helpful frameworks for explaining group dynamics.

According to social exchange theory, individuals join a working group because of the perceived benefits that may be derived from membership. These benefits may be either material or nonmaterial and may include opportunities for social support, professional advancement, help in solving problems, or possibilities of gaining status and/or prestige. Although groups provide opportunities for individuals to obtain these benefits, certain behaviors that contribute to the accomplishment of the goals of the group are expected in return. Thus, an interdependent relationship is formed between each member and the group as a whole. This exchange relationship is characterized as follows. Each member contributes specific skills to a group in return for benefits that are of interest to that member. Each member of the group has skills that can be contributed. Some of these skills are more valuable that others in helping the group achieve their goals. However, all members have something of value to contribute. Each member expects a benefit commensurate with his/her contribution. The group is functioning at maximum capability when exchanges are equitable. That is, the group is most effective when its goals match those of each individual, and the group provides the desired benefits to each member in exchange for that member's skill and contributions.

In determining whether an exchange is equitable, individuals either implicitly or explicitly assess the group situation in terms of three questions:

1. Will I benefit by participating in this group?

2. Can I satisfy group requirements?

3. Are the benefits offered worth the effort?

For individuals to answer these questions in the affirmative, a group climate or a "culture of collaboration" must exist. This culture is characterized by a team approach that supports flexibility and promotes mutual trust, open communication, and cooperation. In an environment of trust and open communication, group members are able to effectively discuss their needs and what they are willing to contribute to the group in exchange for meeting these needs. The following discussion describes how these questions might be approached.

1. *Will I benefit by participating in this group?*

One of the initial questions an individual must ask him or herself is whether there is a personal benefit for participating in a group. This question is one that is continually asked throughout the collaborative process. In joining a group, each individual has an initial sense of what he or she expects to gain from the project (or the benefits of membership), and an idea of what he or she is willing to commit to the project in return for these benefits. For example, a novice researcher may join a group in order to learn research skills and to gain prestige in working with established investigators (benefits). In exchange he or she is willing to conduct literature reviews and to collect Letters of Support (commitment). Therefore, group interactions are initially characterized by a process of negotiation and renegotiation in which there is a successive series of compromises and modifications in participants' ideas, approaches to problem solving, commitments, and benefits. In these group meetings, individuals refine their understanding of the benefits they hope to gain, and based on this understanding, make a decision as to the level of commitment that will be given to the project.

2. *Can I satisfy group requirements?*

A second important question that an individual must ask him/herself whether it is possible to carry out what the group expects. In order for a member of a group to feel confident that he or she can accomplish the tasks necessary to receive the desired benefits, an individual must have a clear idea of what is expected. This requires the group and its leader to define the expectations of the project clearly, so that each member knows the actions that will be necessary and their specific roles. Through open discussion and negotiation, the roles of members become differentiated and members must clearly understand their responsibilities. If each member contributes to the total group effort by doing what he or she is personally best suited to do, and if each group member has clear expectations about what the other members are going to do and how his or her own efforts fit together with theirs, then not only will the skills of each individual be maximized, but each member will have confidence that their efforts will not be wasted.

3. *Are the benefits offered worth the effort?*

Throughout group meetings and exchanges, individuals evaluate whether the benefits they expect to receive are worth their effort. Numerous factors are considered in evaluating the value of a potential benefit. The time commitment required to obtain the benefit, one's compatibility with other group members, and the fit between one's own personal goals and those of the group are just some of the criteria a person may use to determine whether his/her effort will be worthwhile.

10.2 ROLES AND RESPONSIBILITIES OF TEAM MEMBERS

The team building literature provides an understanding of the roles and responsibilities that evolve in a collaborative work effort. These roles are different than those traditionally assumed in working groups. Two concepts are helpful in understanding the roles and responsibilities of team members: role differentiation and role release.

1. *Role Differentiation*—Developing specific and clearly defined roles is a critical aspect of the collaborative group process. It is important for the group to define key roles early in the group process and match the requirements of a particular role with the level of expertise of an individual member. For example, some members are good at curriculum development, others at conducting literature reviews or scientific writing, while still others have expertise in statistics. This process results in specialization of function and increased group stability. Groups operate more effectively when members are assigned tasks that they can do well. Group stability is enhanced under these conditions because uncertainty is reduced when each member is clear about what is expected of him or herself and of others. Unclear roles and poorly defined areas of responsibility ultimately lead to group conflict and dissatisfaction of individuals. Since task requirements of the group change over time, negotiation and renegotiation regarding whom does what and when, is a continuous process.

   Despite its importance, role differentiation can be difficult to achieve. For example, a group leader or another member of the group may assume too much responsibility. This can be as negative as assuming too little responsibility since it leaves others in the group unsure of how to effectively participate. Obtaining just the right balance between individual and group goals involves constant evaluation and monitoring of the group process, the roles that become differentiated, and individual role performance.

2. *Role Release*—Another important aspect of a collaborative effort is that the specific knowledge and expertise of a role is shared with the group in such a way that others can learn the requirements of that role. This practice,

which has been called "role release," is different from that which occurs in an individual or consultative model (Lyon & Lyon, 1980). In these models, an individual or consultant provides expertise to solve a particular problem. However, they do not necessarily share their knowledge or teach others how to solve the problem. In a collaborative team, role release allows members to learn and develop new areas of expertise. This process increases the competence of the group and serves as a way to help individual members develop additional skills.

For example, in a collaborative effort to submit a grant application, one member of the team may assume responsibility for developing a comprehensive review of the literature. This individual would then be responsible for sharing how the search is conducted, the rationale for selecting specific literature, and the specific aspects of the review that are critical for all members to know and understand. In other words, he or she must release or share specific information and knowledge so that the group as a whole develops the same level of expertise. Another member's role might be to develop the budget for the project and obtain the necessary institutional approval prior to the submission of the application. This individual would be responsible for sharing the rationale for the budget and the specific procedural steps involved in developing and obtaining approval so that other members can gain such expertise.

Role differentiation and role release are two key components of a collaborative group structure that facilitate mentoring and professional growth. Team members with little expertise or professional experience in submitting a grant or conducting research are able to make meaningful contributions to the effort through role differentiation and additional skills taught through role release. The opportunity for personal growth is an important benefit of group participation.

3. *Emergent Roles on a Collaborative Team*—There are a number of roles that individuals can assume on a collaborative team. The specific roles that are developed necessarily reflect the content of the grant, the scope of project-related activities, and the areas of expertise of team members.

You may be familiar with the traditional roles that individuals typically assume on a research project as summarized in Table 10-1.

TABLE 10-1   Roles on a Traditional Research Project Structure

Role	Responsibility
Principal Investigator	• Oversees entire project • Contributes discrete area of content expertise • Responsible for scientific integrity of the project
Co-Investigator	• Contributes discrete area of content expertise
Project Coordinator/Director	• Responsible for day-to-date management of the project
Interviewers	• Conducts assessment of subjects or collects data
Interventionist	• Implements experimental protocol in intervention studies
Data Coders/Cleaners	• Cleans data • Checks for accuracy of data entry
Database Manager	• Establishes and maintains data files
Statistician	• Assists in determining statistical analysis

Traditionally, the principal investigator on a research grant assumes major responsibility for establishing the administrative structure, guiding the conceptualization of the project and assuring its scientific integrity. A project director assumes similar responsibilities for an educational program. A co-investigator is primarily responsible for more specialized areas of knowledge, such as theoretical or conceptual contributions, or supervising the implementation of a particular component of a study. The project manager, coordinator, or director is the individual who assumes responsibility for the day-to-day management of a project. This may include screening potential subjects, coordination and scheduling of interviews, supervision of interviewers, assistance in questionnaire development, and management of coding and cleaning of data. Other roles listed on Table 10-1 are associated with the management of data. These include establishing and maintaining a database for statistical analysis, cleaning raw data files, providing statistical assistance, and generating analyses.

There are numerous other roles in a collaborative effort that complement the traditional project structure and facilitate the participation of individuals who may be less experienced in the research process. These roles and associated areas of responsibility are summarized in Table 10-2. This list of roles and responsibilities is not inclusive, but merely suggestive of the way in which multiple tasks can be organized to match the area and level of experience of individual members with the requirements of the group. Each member may assume one or more roles. Effective grant writing teams tend to be most effective with three to six participants. These roles enable individuals with different areas and levels of expertise to participate as equals on a team, since equality of participation is a critical characteristic of a collaborative work effort. Matching specific roles to the area of interest and level of expertise of each member occurs at a group meeting in which members openly discuss what needs to be accomplished, who will assume what responsibility and the time frame for the completion of the task.

As you can see from this table, there are a number of roles that might be assumed by members of a project team at both the proposal writing stage and the implementation stage. The determination of who will carry out what activity depends on the areas of expertise and interests of the team members, and should be negotiated early in the planning process for a grant application.

In addition to the roles listed in Table 10-2, one person needs to assume the role of group leader. The group leader of a collaborative effort has a distinct role on the team, which requires specific group facilitation skills in addition to the technical skills needed to carry out the project. This person may be the principal investigator of a research project or the project director of a training/education grant, or another individual who is appointed to

TABLE 10-2   Roles on a Collaborative Research Team: Primary Responsibilities

Role	Project Development	Implementation
Administrative	• Organize meetings • Record project decisions	• Develop codebooks • Organize and maintain data records
Funding Specialist	• Identify funding sources • Contact agencies • Obtain application	• Serve as contact for agency • Monitor required reports
Subject Specialist	• Organize literature search • Summarize literature	• Review new literature • Conduct periodic searches
Design Expert	• Develop design components	• Monitor implementation
Statistical Expert	• Design statistical approach	• Conduct statistical analyses
Clinical Site Expert	• Represent resources and limitations of site • Design study procedures to fit site	• Monitor procedures • Troubleshoot problems on site • Track patient census
Subject Recruiter	• Identify subject pool • Design recruitment approach	• Conduct or monitor recruitment
Data Collector	• Identify data collection instruments	• Conduct or monitor interviews or data collection
Intervention Expert	• Assist in developing intervention protocol	• Conduct or monitor intervention

coordinate the team effort because of his or her special area of expertise. The group leader must assume overall direction of the collaborative team building effort, as well as facilitate or coordinate the work tasks of the group. He or she must carefully work to build an effective team in which equality of participation is encouraged and shared leadership for the accomplishment of specific work efforts emerges.

Who should be a group leader? This individual should have knowledge of the grantsmanship process in addition to skills in working with groups. He or she must also be willing to commit more time and effort than other members of the team because evaluating and managing the group processes inherent in team development is a time consuming process. The group leader may be appointed by a group or may be the initiator of the team itself. Table 10-3 lists five unique responsibilities of the leader of a collaborative team effort.

TABLE 10-3   Five Group Leader/Facilitator Responsibilities

- Assure that each member is engaged in the group process
- Coordinate the work effort
- Guide the team through each step of the grant submission process
- Serve as mentor, role model as well as group participant
- Recognize when to direct group interactions and when to relinquish control to another team member

10.3 FIVE-STAGE MODEL OF COLLABORATION

Now that you have a basic understanding of the processes that occur in a collaborative effort, let's examine how these processes unfold as a group develops. We have developed a five-stage process model to help guide the development of a collaborative organizational structure. This model, which is illustrated in Figure 1, has been described in detail elsewhere (Gitlin, Lyons & Kolodner, 1994). It was developed to facilitate an interdisciplinary approach to developing and implementing research and education grant programs, and to bridge the gaps between health professionals, practitioners, and researchers.

This process model is based on the principles of social exchange theory and the team building literature and proposes a series of activities that occur in five, purposely implemented overlapping stages. As graphically displayed in Figure 10-1, these are as follows: 1) assessment and goal setting, where key participants examine their individual and institutional goals and assess the need for developing a collaborative relationship, 2) determination of a collaborative fit, where participants discuss and negotiate project ideas and roles, 3) identification of resources and reflection, where participants return to their respective sites to reassess their resources and decide whether to participate, 4) refinement and implementation of the project, where an idea and individual roles are adjusted based on the outcomes of the third stage, and 5) evaluation and feedback, where participants analyze team practices, roles, and establish future goals.

Let's first consider a hypothetical situation in a typical college of health professions presented in Box 10-1 to see how this model can be applied to the development of a project.

BOX 10-1

Dr. L. is an associate professor and clinical coordinator in a department of occupational therapy. In visits to rehabilitation facilities, she notices what appears to be a common theme among therapists working with older patients. The therapists express the concern that many older patients seem resistant or unmotivated in therapeutic sessions. They question whether a better understanding of the aging process would improve their treatment approaches.

Dr. L. reviews the curriculum in her program and is surprised to learn there is minimal content on the aging process. She mentions this to her colleague, Dr. K., in physical therapy, and finds that he has encountered a similar gap between the needs of the therapeutic community and the curriculum. Dr. L. and Dr. K. discover that Ms. G., in nursing, has the same concern. The three coordinators meet and decide to approach this problem by developing an interdisciplinary training grant involving participation of each program. They also decide that involvement of the clinical community in planning the project is critical.

Stage 1: Assessment and goal setting

The scenario above describes the processes that occur in Stage 1. In Stage 1, individuals must first develop an area of interest or concern that needs to be explored with others. In the above scenario, Drs. K. and L., and Ms. G. each independently identified a similar area of concern and interest in aging. Each also understood the importance of geriatric rehabilitation for their profession, department, and institution.

The second task in this stage is to identify potential collaborators. This task was easily accomplished in that the clinical coordinators knew each other and could informally discuss common concerns. In another context, it may involve considerable time and effort to identify potential collaborators, clinical sites, and mutual areas of interest.

Table 10-4 presents six self-study questions to help guide one's thinking in Stage 1.

TABLE 10-4   Self-Study Questions

1. What clinical research and/or educational issues are stimulating and important to me?
2. How do my interests and research/education ideas fit with the goals and priorities of my profession, department, and institution?
3. What expertise and resources are currently in place to develop my area of interest or specific idea?
4. What expertise and resources would be necessary to develop a strong project in this area?
5. What is my level of commitment in terms of time, energy, and other resources to such a project? What is the extent of the commitment I can expect from my department and institution?
6. How willing am I to work with others to shape, develop, and implement this idea?
   a. Am I willing to be flexible and see different sides of a question?
   b. Am I willing to let go of or modify an important idea to fit the interests of others?
   c. Am I willing and able to commit the time to a project?

Stage 2: Determining a collaborative fit

Stage 2 of the model involves two phases and requires that individuals interested in participating come together in a series of meetings to determine if there is a "collaborative fit" and establish an initial commitment to work together. The early phase of this stage involves an evaluation of mutual goals and individual commitment to participation and shared responsibility for project outcomes. If there is agreement on the potential for collaborating in the early phase of this stage, then further discussions and negotiations can proceed. The later phase of this stage is characterized by role differentiation, a clear statement of goals and expectations, and an emerging group structure. A climate of trust will emerge if the negotiations are conducted honestly, if communication is open, if individuals cooperate with one another, and if effective conflict resolution strategies are used. If there is not a collaborative fit, then the project may be abandoned at either phase or a decision may be made to pursue a cooperative or consultative model. Groups that effectively incorporate the viewpoints of others and develop a culture of collaboration will then proceed to Stages 3 and 4.

In the scenario presented in Box 10-1, the three clinical coordinators met to discuss their common area of concern and determine whether they were able to work together to develop and implement a project. They also discussed their own working relationships, personal goals for the year, and the amount of time they had available. Since all three had worked together on projects in the past, they were confident that they could work together on this one. They also agreed that they would keep an open mind about the direction of the project and make sure that it remained relevant to all disciplines.

Stage 3: Resource identification

Stage 3 activities overlap with those of Stage 2. Teams move back and forth between the stages until agreements on major issues and dimensions of the project are reached. That is, having determined that a collaborative fit is possible in Stage 2, participants must return to their respective sites or departments to reflect on the project, identify what they can contribute, and

determine the individual and department advantages of participation. This resource identification and reflection is then brought
back to the group for further discussion. The information from
each respective site may modify the group's initial plans or help
refine its direction.

In the case example, the three members were able to identify resources in each of their departments, such as introductory
course units on aging and faculty recognition of the need to
increase the emphasis. Ms. G., who did not have a doctoral
degree, believed that working with more experienced team members would enhance her skills. Based on their independent
assessments, they realized, however, that they lacked knowledge
of many of the day-to-day practical problems faced by clinicians
and that this knowledge would be critical to a successful curriculum project. Based on these discussions, each team member
contacted a clinical supervisor in one of their affiliated sites, discussed their plan to write a proposal for a training grant and
asked if there was an interest in collaboration. Although each
clinician was excited about the opportunity, they first needed to
discuss their participation and the extent of their efforts with their
department head.

The next step for the team was to confer with their chairmen
to see if the project was desirable for the department and to obtain
release time to work on the grant proposal. Ms. G. learned that her
department was expanding its undergraduate program and this
would require a significant increase in her time to coordinate student clinical experiences. Therefore, this compromised Ms. G.'s
original intent to commit a large portion of her time to the development of the proposal. When she brought this information to the
group for discussion, the group realized that the expansion of the
nursing program actually created new opportunities for their
efforts. However, they also realized that they would need to modify the original plans and role assignments to accommodate Ms.
G.'s time limitations.

Stage 4: Refinement and implementation of project

In Stage 4, the actual work of the proposal writing begins. As the
writing progresses, roles may be refined and procedures redefined.
It is important in this stage to maintain open communication and
handle conflicts or major differences in opinion in an honest and

straightforward manner. Proposal writing can be stressful, especially as deadlines near. Therefore, developing a climate where people help and trust each other will lessen the effects of this stress. Although Murphy's Law, "If anything can go wrong, it will," is usually operative, the other axiom also holds, and that is, "Proposals are always completed on time."

In our example, during Stage 4, the three faculty members met to confer about the structure of the project. They also invited representatives from the rehabilitation facilities to discuss how these organizations would be involved. As the discussion proceeded they found that, in the literature of each of their disciplines, the aging process was covered, but from different perspectives. This literature also suggested different approaches to dealing with the geriatric client. By learning about each other's disciplines, the group was able to identify common themes. They decided to focus on these commonalities to see if, by modifying certain practices, a program could be developed that would be appropriate for all three disciplines. As these ideas evolved, they asked the clinical supervisors to evaluate the potential for success. After a series of meetings, they were able to construct a model program that incorporated ideas from all three disciplines, and actually went beyond what any one discipline offered. It was at this point that they realized that they had developed a very close working relationship and began to feel more like a team than a group.

The team's next task was to determine how they would approach the writing of the proposal. They each discussed their strengths and experiences. They agreed that, since the initial idea for the project was Dr. L.'s, she would take the lead and coordinate the proposal writing activities and have responsibility for contacting the funding agency. Dr. K. volunteered to serve as editor, especially for the final draft and develop the budget in collaboration with Dr. L. Ms. G. agreed to obtain the letters of support and gather the references, which can be time consuming. She also offered to have the secretary in her department take responsibility for final typing, formatting, and developing time lines and other graphics. They also agreed to conduct a thorough literature search in their own disciplines, write a draft of a section of the proposal, and obtain letters of support from contacts in their discipline.

During the negotiations and discussion of the details of the project, a number of disagreements occurred. However, Dr. L., in her role as team coordinator, identified areas for which there was agreement and checked for consensus at key points in the discussion. She also reminded everyone that it was important that all concerns about any aspect of the project be brought to the team's attention. All concerns were given a full and open hearing as the group worked toward obtaining consensus. The writing of the proposal was completed the day before the due date. During the last day each member of the team had specific responsibilities for putting the final touches on the application. For example, Dr. K. reviewed the final draft for consistency and completeness, Ms. G. supervised the duplication of the required number of copies, and Dr. L. delivered the application to the post office that evening.

Stage 5: Evaluation and feedback

Once the proposal is completed, the entire process needs to be evaluated by all team members. Evaluation and feedback is an essential component of each stage of the model, which we discuss in the next section. However, Stage 5 represents a formal evaluation of the entire process by all team members. This evaluation should assess team functioning and include an honest reflection on the way members communicated, resolved conflicts, and made decisions. Table 10-5 presents a list of six questions to help guide this evaluation. The assessment is a very important component of a collaborative model. It not only provides an evaluation of how well the group functioned, but also prepares the team to engage in future collaborative efforts. If the proposal is funded, the group will also have the responsibility of carrying out the project, and this assessment will help them improve their ability to function as a team in the future.

In our example, the team decided to wait two weeks after the proposal was mailed before meeting again to assess the proposal writing process. They believed that this period of time was long enough to allow them to "catch their breath," and yet still close enough to the experience so that the strengths and weaknesses of the process would be fresh in everyone's minds.

TABLE 10-5   Evaluation of Team Effectiveness

---

1. Are there clear, cooperative goals to which every member has been committed?
2. Has there been accurate and effective communication of ideas and feelings?
3. Has there been distributed participation and leadership?
4. Were decision-making procedures appropriate and effective?
5. Did controversy and differences of opinion lead to productive solutions?
6. Is there evidence of high levels of trust, acceptance, support among members and a high level of cohesion?

10.4 INDICATORS OF COLLABORATION

How do you know if your group is effectively progressing and evolving into a collaborative team? What are the indicators that a culture of collaboration is emerging? The development of teams through the use of the five-stage model involves conscious recognition of group processes and the purposeful shaping of exchanges to nurture the emergence of collaboration. At each stage of the model, there are specific indicators that suggest the group is progressing effectively. These indicators are the 14 characteristics described in chapter 9. The specific stage in which they are expected to emerge are shown in Table 10-6.

Monitoring these indicators at group meetings is an important activity that can be used to facilitate the emergence of a culture of collaboration. This process may occur informally when the group leader and/or one or two other group members discuss the progress of the team. It also may occur more formally when an objective evaluator observes the group process and its outcomes, or it may occur by using a combination of informal and formal techniques.

Informal Evaluation: An informal assessment merely entails reflecting on the interactions at meetings and recording the group's strengths and weaknesses. Using this approach, the leader and one or more team members briefly meet after each team

TABLE 10-6   Stage, Task, and Indicators of Effectiveness

Stage	Task	Primary Indicators of Effective Team Effort
1	Assessment and Goal Setting	• Mutual or shared goals • Clear statement of goals, expectations, and procedures
2	Determination of a Collaborative Fit (Early phase)	• Cooperation • Open, honest negotiation • Climate of trust being established • Shared decision-making
2	Determination of a Collaborative Fit (Later phase)	• Open communication • Role differentiation • Conflict resolution
3	Resource Identification and Reflection	• Equality of participation • Shared responsibility for participation
4	Project Refinement and Implementation	• Shared leadership • Group cohesion • Decision-making by consensus
5	Evaluation	Three levels of assessment • Individual • Group • External observer

meeting to evaluate the group interactions and assess them using the 14 indicators of collaboration. It is helpful to simply record those aspects of the group meeting that represent a "green light" or a "red flag." "Green lights" are those interactions that signal that the group has reached a level of consensus and cohesion and is ready to move ahead. "Red flags" are those interactions that suggest major differences persist among group members. For example, in Stage 1, a "green light" may be that all team members appear to be actively engaged in the discussion and are able to articulate specific project goals that are consistent, an indicator that "mutual goals" can be achieved. A "red flag" in this stage may be that members indicate limited time to commit or introduce widely conflicting approaches to developing the project. Recognition of interactions that indicate "green lights" or "red flags" enables the leader to structure interactions that can move the team forward. In conducting an informal assessment, it is important to identify particular behaviors or statements that illustrate a green light or that are indicative of the characteristics of collaboration for that stage. For example, by the conclusion of Stage 1, the expectation is that members agree on a set of broad project goals that are clearly articulated. Box 10-2 illustrates an interaction that reflects two indicators that a positive collaborative relationship is forming; expression of mutual goals, and clear statement of expectations and procedures.

BOX 10-2

Ms. K.: "I am interested in pursuing a project that will advance assessment of the physical home environment. An objective assessment would enable us to provide comprehensive and effective home modifications to our clients."

Dr. L.: "I agree. Let's structure a project to develop an assessment tool and evaluate its psychometric properties. This would benefit both the researcher and health provider."

Dr. J.: "This might be difficult to accomplish. We may need to consult with an expert in questionnaire design. But I agree, this should be our primary goal."

This interaction represents a "green light." That is, members appear committed to pursuing a joint project and there is agreement as to its nature and scope. In this case, the group leader can move the group to the next stage of team development that would involve discussion of the details of the project and potential funding opportunities.

Consider, on the other hand, the interaction in Box 10-3 that raises a "red flag."

In this interaction, the group is not ready to advance its work. Although members of the group have agreed on an area of mutual interest (delirium in the elderly in acute care hospital settings), the way to proceed (research vs. training project) remains unresolved.

This represents a basic disagreement, and a potentially serious conflict. There is no evidence of a clear statement of group goals or direction at this point in the group's discussion. In this case, the group leader needs to have the group gather more information and then meet again to determine if this difference in approach can be resolved. The leader may assign each member a task. For example, one member might be asked to conduct a literature review of research and training of health professional in delirium. Another member might be asked to identify potential research and training funding sources in this area. The group will remain in the early phase of Stage 1 until they can reach a mutually agreeable solution as to the nature and scope of the project.

BOX 10-3

Dr. S.: "I agree that delirium is a serious problem that we often see with the elderly who enter the acute care setting. But we do not, as of yet, know the best practices for minimizing this problem. Therefore, I suggest we focus on describing and evaluating current practices as one approach to determine what works."

Dr. M: "But this problem is so pervasive. I would like to develop training materials immediately to enable practitioners to work with the elderly more effectively."

Ms. B: "But what would these training materials include? Don't we first need to study the issue and see what is out there?"

Dr. M: "No. I disagree. That would take too long. We could develop a consensus panel to establish training materials and than train health practitioners within the year."

Formal Evaluation: You might also consider a formal evaluative approach that involves a systematic evaluation from three perspectives: 1) an appraisal of the nature of group interactions, 2) each member's appraisal of their own behavior in the group and 3) each member's appraisal of the other members' behaviors in the group. The triangulation of three perspectives provides an understanding of the extent to which collaboration and group cohesiveness exists.

In a formal approach, an external reviewer is hired or a member of the group agrees to serve as the evaluator. The evaluator must remain an objective observer of group interactions. The evaluator may want to observe and record specific behaviors that illustrate the 14 indicators of a collaborative project structure. We have developed evaluative questions to guide how to identify these 14 indicators (see appendix C). Additionally, we recommend that the evaluator systematically obtain appraisals from individuals as to the group process which can be used at the conclusion of Stages 2 and 4 (see appendix C).

The evaluator's role is also to provide feedback to the group. The purpose of this is to strengthen team building. By identifying behaviors that promote positive team performance, group members can consciously strive to model effective team building behaviors and advance team functioning. Box 10-4 provides one example of the way constructive feedback can be provided to a team to strengthen its efforts.

An evaluative process can also combine formal and informal approaches. Evaluation is an important reflective activity that helps each member clarify his or her own personal goals and can significantly advance the efforts of the group. Some form of evaluation must occur at each stage of the model.

10.5 COMMON PROBLEMS IN COLLABORATIVE TEAMS AND EFFECTIVE SOLUTIONS

Group work is a dynamic process that involves continual negotiation and renegotiation of goals and the roles and responsibilities of each group member. Since these efforts occur over time, groups are in a constant state of flux and change. As a consequence, a number of difficulties may emerge in the process of collaborating as groups move through the five stages of the collaborative model. These problems may concern either individual members, the dynamics of the group or changes at the institutional level. Table 10-7 summarizes some common problems in collaborative group work and solutions that are effective.

BOX 10-4

EVALUATION FEEDBACK

I have observed five group meetings and have asked each member to complete two questionnaires. Let me begin by discussing my observations of the team's performance. First, it has been very exciting to see how the group's commitment to its goals has emerged over this period of time. This is evident in that each team member comes to the meetings on time and actively participates in the discussions. Also, there is strong evidence of respect for each member's opinion and there appears to be equality of participation. By this I mean that each person has at one point or another taken responsibility for steering the group back on track when discussions deviate, and that individuals appear to feel comfortable enough to challenge expressed opinions or at least ask for clarification.

One point I would like to emphasize is that the group has not yet clearly differentiated roles and responsibilities of members. That is, each member appears to be still unclear as to his or her specific responsibilities and tasks. This is evident from the responses on the questionnaires in which most members responded that they had not been assigned specific areas of responsibility and were unclear as to their specific roles. It is also evident in my own observations. For example, there appears to be confusion about the responsibilities of the group leader. On several occasions the group leader has asked for assistance in carrying out particular tasks and no one readily volunteered. The group leader in turn has expressed feeling burdened due to assuming more of the workload than is reasonable.

I recommend that the group spend some time at this meeting discussing each person's expectations about their specific roles and responsibilities as well as that of the group leader. Also, the group might want to discuss a more effective way of assigning tasks. It is important to clarify roles especially at this juncture, since the group needs to accomplish many tasks in a timely fashion during the next month.

TABLE 10-7   Common Problems and Solutions

Common Problems	*Possible Solutions*
I. INDIVIDUAL MEMBERS	
1. Divisive working behaviors which impede group work	• Reexamine personal goals and team goals • Restate main goals and objectives • Establish ground rules for interaction • Facilitate healthy disagreement
2. Time lines not being met	• Renegotiate roles, responsibilities, and expectations • Identify barriers to completing tasks on time • Establish open communications to facilitate task completion • Develop contingency plans
3. Individual changes in priorities/goals	• Renegotiate roles on team • Expand areas of responsibility when appropriate • Be prepared from outset for changes in expectations and personal goals • Be prepared for a member to leave the group and for others to join
II. GROUP INTERACTION	
1. Conflict/differences in opinion on how to proceed	• Allow all differences to be discussed • State main goal and objective of the team • Work through each conflicting position to see if they meet team objectives • Obtain opinion of expert outside of the group to inform group decisions
2. Use of different vocabulary and way of conceptulizations of an issue	• Have team jointly review key articles that outline concepts • Discuss implications of different approaches • Ensure final decisions are stated clearly
3. Unclear goals; group seems to drift, lose sense of purpose	• Keep running record of group decisions • Start each meeting by reviewing what has been accomplished and what still needs to be done

(continued)

Common Problems	*Possible Solutions*
III. INSTITUTION-RELATED	
1. Priorities/goals of participating institution change	• Team needs to be prepared for change in working environment • Anticipate shifts in goals by keeping each member informed • Assign members specific responsibilities which involve keeping abreast of institutional changes

Individual-based Problems: There are a number of difficulties that may arise in a collaborative team effort that are related to the behaviors of individual members. Behaviors of individuals, such as dominating discussions, interrupting other members before they have an opportunity to complete a statement, ridiculing ideas, or taking a negative approach to the project are not uncommon, especially in the beginning stage of collaboration. Some individuals are just not ready for collaboration. They may be threatened by the group process, may not endorse the goals of the group, may lack appropriate group skills, or may have a personal agenda that differs from the goals of the group. These behaviors cause divisiveness and prevent the development of group cohesion. The group needs to establish ground rules for behavior, which assure that divisive behaviors are not tolerated. The group leader will need to take control of meetings and redirect the group by not permitting an individual to dominate, by modeling expected behaviors, and by clearly reinforcing the value of each member's ideas.

The leader may also consider using a structured brainstorming session to demonstrate the advantages of team problem solving over individual solutions, emphasize that the participation of each member is valued, and assist the group in arriving at a consensus as to the goals of a project. Box 10-5 describes one approach to structuring a brainstorming session.

Here are the *rules* to follow for a brainstorming session:

Part One: Identifying Topics or Ideas

1. Let's say that an academic department is trying to develop an integrated program of research. The department chair or group leader begins by stating the problem area

BOX 10-5

WHAT IS A BRAINSTORMING SESSION?

Brainstorming is a problem-solving technique that enables a group to think outside the box and generate a number of ideas. In brainstorming, each individual suspends criticism or evaluation until all ideas have been exhausted. Each idea that is presented is considered valid and, initially, the purpose is to generate as many ideas as possible.

to be discussed in general terms. For example, the leader might start with the statement, "Our first task is to identify broad topic areas of research that we might want to pursue. Examples of broad topic areas include: health promotion among culturally diverse populations; oral self-care practices among poor rural elderly; or oral health of individuals with AIDS."

2. Each participant spends *five* minutes writing down a list of research topics or specific research questions within these broad areas that interest them.

3. Participants are then encouraged to set aside their analytic and reasoning mind and approach the process in a spontaneous way.

4. A basic ground rule at this stage is that any research topic or question for investigation is valid. This session is "free-wheeling" and all ideas are accepted without any evaluative remarks (either critical or humorous).

5. One participant is appointed as the recorder and, using a flip chart or blackboard, records each idea.

6. Each participant, in order, states the first topic area on their sheet.

7. This process is repeated until all the ideas of each participant have been recorded.

8. Each idea is recorded in order of presentation. All ideas that are expressed are recorded without any evaluation.

9. At the end of this session, the group will have generated a lengthy list of potential research areas for investigation.

Part Two: Prioritizing Ideas

1. Once the list of topics is complete, participants must then begin to categorize and prioritize these ideas. The first task is to group topics into similar areas. For example, all topics that are related to community-based interventions, or all topics that are related to health promotion should be grouped together. The second task is to prioritize each topic as either those of immediate interest or those of potential interest to all team members.

2. For those topics that are prioritized as of "immediate interest," participants should discuss the specific aspects of the topic that would be of interest to pursue. For example, members are asked to answer the following question:

    "What about this topic, _____, is of interest/importance?"

3. It is at this point in the session that ideas are "massaged" and evaluated, and participants bring their analytic selves back to the discussion. Each idea is evaluated critically as to its feasibility in addition to its interest to group members.

4. At the end of this session, the group should have three to five topic areas and specific research questions for each. It is important that this process not be hurried. If it becomes clear that more discussion is needed to reach agreement on the topic areas, schedule a second meeting for this discussion.

The group leader has a responsibility not only to ensure that this process is followed, but also to monitor and prevent divisive behaviors. In this way, brainstorming serves two purposes. It helps identify topics for investigation, which the entire team can agree on, and it sets a tone for the group that defines acceptable and unacceptable behavior. This activity also reinforces the value of equality of participation and places equal value on each idea. Finally, the group learns quickly that the list produced by the entire team is more comprehensive and sophisticated than that of any one individual.

A second common problem in collaborative work is that a team member may have difficulty completing a task by the expected time. Other responsibilities or changes in personal priorities may take precedence for that individual. Although this may inadvertently happen to anyone, the inability to meet a deadline may have serious consequences for other members of a team, especially when a grant application must be completed by a designated date. Therefore, it is important to assure that all tasks are accomplished in a timely fashion. Strategies that can be used include circulating a written list of the tasks agreed upon and the expected date of their completion to team members, developing contingency plans for completing difficult tasks, or renegotiating the roles and areas of responsibility of individual members to assure that all tasks can be completed. It is the responsibility of the group leader to periodically check the progress of each team member in completing these assigned tasks.

Another common occurrence in group work is that individual priorities and personal goals change with time. Individuals may leave a group or seek different roles within it. A group needs to be prepared for shifts in the composition of the team and be ready to engage in negotiations regarding changing role responsibilities.

Group-based problems: The dynamics of a group itself may pose its own set of difficulties or potential barriers to team success. A natural part of group interaction is the expression of differences of opinion that can be either positive or negative. On the positive side, differences of opinion stimulate thinking and can point out inconsistencies or lack of clarity in the group's approach. If dealt with in a positive manner, differences can result in more creative ideas. On the negative side, they can be a potential source of disruption. It is important, therefore, to allow differences in perspectives and opinions to be discussed openly and evaluate how these discussions strengthen or contribute toward the main goal and objective of the team.

A second potential problem is that individuals from different disciplines enter the group with distinct work styles, a specialized vocabulary, and diverse ways of conceptualizing problems. As the group works together it is important to build a common vocabulary and to understand how each discipline conceptualizes ideas and problems. Once a common base is developed, it allows the group to integrate diverse ideas and build beyond what each discipline can contribute separately. One way to build a common foundation is to have team members read the same set of articles that examine the problem area from different perspectives. This provides members with an understanding of different approaches and vocabularies. Vocabulary and conceptual approaches must be discussed by the team and an agreement must be reached about the common language that will be used.

A third common problem is that a group may seem to lose its sense of direction or purpose. This may occur if discussions become redundant or during periods when there is little to do. To keep a group on track, a running record of group decisions and a review of these decisions at the beginning of each meeting is helpful. Another strategy is to stop meeting for a period of time. If there is no reason to meet, there should be no meeting. For example, if a group is meeting weekly during periods of intense activity, then during low periods, a better use of time might be to meet on a less frequent basis, such as once a month.

Institutional-based Problems: Another potential source of difficulties which may impede group performance is institutional. The priorities or goals of a department or institution may change due to a new department head or dean with a different philosophy, institutional reorganization, or changes in financial stability. Often there is very little that a group can do to overcome these changes. However, if the group has developed a culture of collaboration, they will have a flexible attitude and be able to accommodate such changes. Sharing information among members keeps everyone appropriately informed of anticipated changes and prepared for change.

SUMMARY

This chapter presented a framework for understanding the process of collaboration.

1. Collaboration has been discussed using the theoretical framework of social exchange theory and literature on team building.

2. In a collaborative structure, there are specific roles and responsibilities for each member of a team. These roles are different than those within a traditional project structure. The concepts of role differentiation and role release are helpful to understand these different roles.

3. A five-stage model of collaboration was presented to effectively guide the development and functioning of a collaborative team. The stages are labeled: assessment and goal setting, determination of a collaborative fit, identification of resources, refinement and implementation, and evaluation and feedback.

4. Evaluation of collaborative teamwork can be accomplished using 14 indicators of a collaborative structure as a guide. This evaluation can be conducted either informally, by members of the team, or more formally, by an outside evaluator.

5. Group work is a dynamic process, influenced by the personalities of members and changes in the institutional environment. As a result, a number of challenges may occur throughout the life of the group. Challenges will emerge that are related to individuals, to the dynamics of the group itself, and to the institution. Successful teams are those that monitor their own functioning and have developed the mechanisms by which to work through common difficulties.

Part V

Life After a Proposal Submission

Yes, there is a life after a proposal submission! After the hard work and hectic pace of submitting an application, you might not want to think about the proposal anymore, or at least for awhile. That is okay, because it will take some time for your proposal to be evaluated and a funding determination made.

But what does happen to your proposal when it leaves your hands? If you were to visit a federal agency in Washington, D.C., on the date that grants are due, you would see the hallways cluttered with stacks of applications. Although it will appear chaotic, there is an organized process by which grant applications are categorized, assigned an identification number, and then sent out to a designated individual to be evaluated.

Knowledge of this process and how applications are reviewed can enhance the quality of your submission. Understanding the review process is an important aspect of grantsmanship and the focus of chapter 11. In this chapter, we describe the grant review process, the criteria used by reviewers to evaluate applications, the potential outcomes of a review, and categories of acceptance and rejection. The worst mistake of new investigators is to feel so overwhelmed by a rejection that the comments of the review panel are not even read. However, there are a number of options if you are not funded. These are also considered in chapter 11. It is important to recognize that few grant applications receive funding on the first submission, so consideration of and planning for a resubmission is a basic aspect of the process of grantsmanship.

Program officers often claim that just by reading proposals, applicants enhance their ability to develop a competitive grant. chapter 12 provides a case study in which we present an excerpt from a proposal and demonstrate how it would be critiqued. In addition to carefully examining chapter 12, try to arrange other opportunities for reading applications and the comments of reviewers, so that you can become more skilled at developing proposals and interpreting reviewers' evaluations.

Chapter 11

Understanding the Review Process

- Structure of the Review Process
- Review Criteria and Categories of Acceptance and Rejection
- Resubmission Options

Once you have mailed or delivered your grant application to a funding agency, take the opportunity to sit back and relax. It may take six to nine months, or sometimes longer depending upon the agency, to learn whether your proposal will be funded. You may wonder what happens to your proposal once it is submitted to an agency. Knowledge of the review enables you to understand and analyze the review score you will receive, as well as helps you prepare a more competitive application, particularly if resubmission is necessary.

Before submitting a proposal to an agency, it is importation to inquire about the process and evaluation criteria that will be used to review applications. Also, you should inquire as to whether names of reviewers are available to the public prior to submission. The NIH publishes a list of members on all its standing review groups and updates this publication yearly. Other agencies such as the Department of Education only release the names of its reviewers at the conclusion of a funding cycle. This is much less helpful since it is difficult to discern the particular competition for which a reviewer participated. Occasionally, foundations provide a list of their reviewers either as part of their annual reports, on their web pages, or upon request. Knowledge of the reviewers' degrees and scientific backgrounds provides insight as to the particular areas of expertise that are represented on a panel. In the NIH system, if you submit a proposal for which special expertise is required and members on the existing scientific review panel do not represent this expertise, you may request, in the form of a letter with your application, that a specialist review your proposal. For competitions in which it is not possible to obtain reviewer names, it is important to try to obtain information about the general background of reviewers. For example, it would be important to know if consumers as well as research scientists will be reviewing your work. This provides insight as to how best to explain your ideas in the proposal so that it is clear to reviewers.

Each agency applies different evaluative criteria in the review process. Furthermore, within an agency, different criteria may be applied for specific competitions that are sponsored. As discussed in chapter 2, usually evaluative criteria are provided as part of the guidelines for submission or within the application kit. It is important to address each of these criteria carefully in your application. For example, one competition may emphasize innovation and significance of the proposed research or education idea, whereas another may emphasize innovation in dissemination and weight this section higher than others. Thus, how you develop your ideas and the level of detail you provide will be influenced by the importance the agency attributes to different sections. Finally, as part of understanding the review process, you should inquire whether an application can be resubmitted if it is not funded on the first review cycle and the number of resubmissions that are permissible. For NIH unsolicited applications, it is possible to submit the same application up to three times. However, this may not be the case for special competitions such as requests for applications (RFA) or in other agencies.

This chapter describes the review process and provides guidelines for interpreting reviewers' comments to help you decide whether to resubmit your application if it is not funded. We also briefly outline your responsibilities once you do receive funding.

11.1 STRUCTURE OF THE REVIEW PROCESS

Each funding agency establishes its own set of procedures from which to conduct a rigorous and comprehensive review of proposals. As noted above, these procedures may differ for each competition sponsored by a particular agency. Whereas foundations tend to establish special review panels or appoint a board that assumes review responsibilities for their competitions, federal agencies follow the procedures discussed here.

Let's examine the general review procedures followed by federal agencies and specifically, the Public Health Service (PHS), which includes the National Institutes of Health and the Agency for Healthcare Research and Quality (AHRQ). The Public Health Service (PHS) has a sequential review process that is referred to as a "dual review system" for investigator- initiated applications (e.g., R01, R03 or other competing applications). First, all applications are sent to a general receiving office called the Center for Scientific Review (CSR), formerly referred to as the Division of Research Grants (DRG). For each funding cycle, over 10,000 applications may be received by the CSR; and in one year over 40,000 applications will be reviewed. At the CSR, more than a dozen staff members, referred to as Referral Officers, assign a referral number to the application and examine .it for completeness. These individuals have extensive expertise in research administration and the review process. Then, on the basis of key words in the title or abstract of the application, the Referral Officers make several assignments. First, they assign proposals to an Institutional Center (IC) that is one of the institutes of the NIH, such as the National Institute on Aging. In your cover letter to the CSR, you should indicate to which Institute you want your proposal assigned (for a list of the NIH institutes see: http://www.nih.gov/icd).

Second, they assign proposals to what is now called an Integrated Review Group (IRG); and then within the IRG, to what is called a study section. This process is referred to as triaging the proposal. There are 19 IRGs, each representing a broad category of research (e.g., Behavioral and Social Science, Oncological Sciences, Pathophysiological Sciences). Each IRG is in turn composed of an average of three to seven study sections. Study sections consist of research scientists who are responsible for reviewing applications for scientific merit. Study section members are selected based on rigorous academic and scholarly standards and are usually appointed for multi-term years. There may be 15 or more individuals per study section. In your cover letter to the CSR, you may request a particular study section that you think is most appropriate for the review of your application (a roster of the study sections can be found at http://www.csr.nih.gov/Committees/rosterindex.asp).

As you can see, the triaging of your proposal is based principally on your title and brief abstract. Thus, it is important for you to carefully construct these aspects of the proposal so it is assigned to the study section best suited to review your application. It can take anywhere from six to eight weeks for these assignments to be made. Once completed, the CSR mails each reviewer a copy of the applications they are to review in that funding cycle. Also, within six to eight weeks following the submission date, you will receive a postcard indicating the following information: a) the IRG assignment; b) the name of the Scientific Review Administrator (SRA); c) the Institute assignment (e.g., National Institute on Aging, National Eye Institute); and d) the number the agency assigned to your proposal for reference and referral. This application receipt is very important and should be filed securely. If you have any questions about your proposal, you will need to use the information provided on this receipt to track it down with the CSR or SRA.

In most federal reviews, study section members are brought together to evaluate proposals for their scientific and technical merit and make a recommendation for funding. Members of the review panel typically have four to eight weeks to review up to 20 or 30 applications. The number of applications varies depending on the agency and particular competition.

Although rare, there are three other operating structures used by federal agencies. For some competitions, reviewers do not receive the applications in advance. Instead, they must travel to Washington, D.C., and stay for about a week of work that involves both independent reading of proposals in a hotel room followed by group meetings. Alternately, for certain competitions, only a small panel is required and sometimes these are conducted by teleconferencing. Occasionally if a special expert is required to review an application, he or she may join through telephone conferencing while the study section is meeting face-to-face.

In each study section, a representative from the funding agency moderates or oversees the deliberations of the review panel. This representative, referred to as the Scientific Review Administrator (SRA) in the PHS system, or as the project officer in the Department of Education, assures that each application receives a fair and thorough review. In preparation for the review, the SRA assures that the application is complete and assigns a reviewer from the standing committee to write up the summary and other members of the study section as readers who must come prepared to discuss the application. In the NIH system, each study section also appoints a "chairperson" from its membership who sits next to the SRA and is responsible for conducting the review meeting. In some agencies, such as HRSA, the SRA appoints not only a primary reviewer, but also a secondary reviewer and, occasionally, a third reviewer. These reviewers are responsible for an in-depth evaluation of the proposal, whereas this is not the expectation for the other members of the review panel who sometimes may only receive the proposal abstract. At the review meetings, the primary reviewer presents a concise description of the proposal, a critique, and a score. The secondary reviewer(s) then add additional points and their score. The third reviewer's comments and score are then presented, followed by a full panel discussion in which members may ask for clarification of points. Each member of the panel is then asked to record their score independently.

Under the new "streamlining procedures" implemented in NIH, one week prior to convening a study section, the SRA obtains a list from study section reviewers of the applications that received initial scores for scientific merit in the lower half of the proposals read (described below). These applications will not be discussed as part of the face-to-face deliberations of the study section, unless, at the time of the meeting, one or more reviewers request that an application be discussed. The applicant will then receive unedited summations from each reviewer but not a percentile score (see below). Although this does not mean that the application is disapproved for funding, it does indicate that the application would not have received a score that would have allowed it to be considered for funding.

During the panel discussion, the SRA may not express an opinion regarding the merits of an application nor assign a score. His or her role is to provide technical assistance, clarify agency policies, and, in some agencies, write a summary of the review for each proposal. This summary statement represents a synthesis of the deliberations of the review panel and includes a description of the proposed project, its areas of strength and weakness, and the rationale for the panel's recommendation, as well as a numeric rating of the proposal. It is this summary, once called the "pink sheets" in the NIH system (because it used to be printed on pink paper), that the investigator receives whether or not he or she receives funding.

Following completion of this level of scientific review, the agency prepares a master list of all the applications reviewed by the panels and their rankings. Also, a summary sheet is prepared for each application that includes each reviewer's comments, a summary of strengths and weakness that highlight discussion points of the panel, and a score. The summary sheets and the ranking of each application are then submitted to the program staff of the IC or assigned Institute of the NIH and to the investigator. In turn, the IC staff refers the list of recommendations for funding to their respective board of individuals who evaluate the decision for funding. In the NIH system, this board is referred to as the "National Advisory Council." The Council is composed of scientists and non-scientists who review each funding recommendation with regard to whether the proposal reflects the overall mission of the agency and the adequacy of protection for human subjects. The National Advisory Council meets three times a year to determine the final funding status of applications. An application must be approved at both levels of the review process, the study section and Council, in order for funding to occur.

In contrast to the NIH system, other divisions of the government, such as the Bureau of Health Professions (BHPr) and Department of Education, do not have standing study sections. These agencies appoint a group of individuals, three to five for the Department of Education and up to 10 or 15 for the BHPr, to serve as reviewers for each competition. Typically, a program officer is responsible for identifying appropriate individuals for review panels. This is a time consuming process in which the program officer must select scientists and sometimes consumers, if specified by legislation, who are not employed by the federal government and who have expertise in the particular area specified for the competition. The program officer must also assure representation from diverse geographic regions and among minority groups. Usually, only one member of an institution can serve on a review panel and in some competitions, it is prohibited to have a panelist from the same state as an applicant.

Let's look at a typical review situation, first using as an example the process for the Department of Education, and then the NIH system.

> Dr. S. is an associate professor at a major university with special expertise in disability research. He agrees to serve on a review panel for the Department of Education that is scheduled to meet in the second week of April. Six weeks prior to the group meeting in Washington, D.C., he receives eight proposals to review, for four of which he is given the responsibility of primary reviewer and for four of which he is a secondary reviewer. He also receives a detailed set of instructions and a comprehensive evaluation sheet that needs to be completed for each proposal.

On those applications for which he is the primary review-er, Dr. S. will need to write a comprehensive description and critique of the project to present during panel deliberations. He will be responsible for representing the application. For example, if a member of the review panel has a question regarding a particular procedure in the application, Dr. S. would be responsible for clarifying the issue based upon his careful reading.

In addition to his responsibilities as a reviewer, Dr. S. has a full teaching load, committee assignments, his own research, and commitments for presentations, manuscripts, and grant applications. Each proposal may need one to three careful readings to provide an adequate evaluation. In order to fulfill all his other obligations, Dr. S. will need to review most of the proposals in the evenings and on weekends if he expects to meet the April deadline. Obviously, Dr. S. is not going to be too happy if a proposal he is reviewing at 10 o'clock in the evening is difficult to read, filled with typographical errors, has sections missing, or omits information which fits the evaluation criteria.

As Dr. S. reviews his set of proposals, he realizes that he is currently a consultant to an institution from which he has received an application. He immediately contacts the agency to notify them of a potential conflict of interest. The agency requests that he return the application and informs Dr. S. that he will have to step out of the room during the panel deliberations for that application.

Dr. S. finishes evaluating the proposals and travels to Washington, D.C., for the panel meeting. He arrives on a Sunday night and participates in an orientation session. On Monday morning, his 10-member panel meets and begins to review a total of 40 proposals. The primary reviewer for each proposal spends about 15 to 20 minutes summarizing the application and providing an evaluation. The secondary reviewer may spend an additional 10 minutes adding his or her comments, areas of disagreement or agreement with the primary reviewer, and his or her evaluation. Other members of the panel after reading the abstract and listening to the two evaluations, then spend about 10 minutes asking questions. Some may have received the application and read it prior to the meeting, while others must make a judgment of merit based upon the primary and secondary reviewers' presentations. As a result of this discussion, the panel decides to approve the proposal. Since this proposal was approved, the panel must then assign it a score and review the budget carefully to determine if modifications are necessary. Upon completion of this discussion, the panel realizes they have spent too much time discussing a controversial aspect of this one proposal and they have 39 applications more to discuss before they can go home. Each member silently hopes that the remaining proposals will not be difficult to review so that they can make fair decisions and still get back home before their children are grown.

Now let's see what happens when Dr. S. reviews for the NIH system.

Dr. S., as a permanent member of a study section, meets with his panel three times a year in Washington, D.C., to review up to 20 or more applications. Of these, he might be assigned as the primary, secondary, or tertiary reviewer for possibly one to eight applications. As with the Department of Education review process, each type of reviewer for the NIH study section has a specific responsibility. As a primary reviewer, Dr. S. responsible for providing both a written and oral presentation that includes a clear, comprehensive, although brief description or overview of the application followed by a detailed critique using the evaluative criteria described below. As a secondary reviewer, he is asked to write a critique and at the meeting to either state agreement or disagreement with the primary reviewer or raise points that were not previously presented. As a tertiary reviewer, Dr. S. asked to write a brief critique and then provide commentary or key points not covered by either the primary or secondary reviewers.

Dr. S. meets with other members of the study section in Washington, D.C., for one and a half to two long days. Each application is allocated 10 to 15 minutes for presentation, discussion, and scoring. Typically, the following procedures are used. The primary, secondary, and tertiary reviewers are first asked to state their score (see scoring ranges below). Then, the primary reviewer presents a summary of the research study and a critique, highlighting strengths and weakness following the five criteria shown below. Following this presentation, the secondary and tertiary reviewers present points that have not been raised. Then a discussion by all panel members ensues. Panel members may ask Dr. S. to clarify points, or may raise other strengths or areas of concern. Dr. S. must be prepared to answer questions about the process, clarify misconceptions, and argue in support of or against an application. In some respects, for those 15 minutes, he is in the hot seat.

If the scores and critiques by the three reviewers are vastly discrepant, the SRA makes a special point of encouraging discussion to reconcile these differences. At the conclusion of the discussion, each reviewer is then asked to restate his or her score taking into consideration the points raised by the panel. They are encouraged to modify their scores particularly when they are extremely divergent in order to derive consensus and a cohesive critique of each application. Following this, in view of the reviewers' presentations and ensuing discussion, each panel member privately scores the application using a scoring sheet provided by the SRA, which is collected at the end of the review.

As you can see, being a reviewer is a time consuming and arduous task. Reviewers have limited time to read and fully comprehend your proposal. Thus, it is very important for you to make it as easy as possible for a reviewer to understand your ideas and plan of action. This is accomplished, in part, by assuring that your writing is clear, that you present your ideas in an organized, concise, and logical manner, and that you check for typographical errors and overall appearance of the application prior to its submission.

11.2 REVIEW CRITERIA

Specific evaluative criteria are used for each grant competition to appraise the scientific and technical merits of proposals. Evaluative criteria differ by agency as well as by type of competition. For investigator-initiated proposals submitted to the NIH system, five standard criteria are used in the review process, as outlined in Box 11-1 (for more detailed information about these criteria and the review process, consult the NIH web site (http://www.drg.nih.gov/guidelines/r01.htm).

BOX 11-1

NIH EVALUATIVE CRITERIA

Significance: Does this study address an important problem? If the aims of the application are achieved, how will scientific knowledge be advanced? What will be the effect of these studies on the concepts or methods that drive this field?

Approach: Are the conceptual framework, design, methods, and analyses adequately developed, well integrated, and appropriate to the aims of the project? Does the applicant acknowledge potential problem areas and consider alternative tactics?

Innovation: Does the project employ novel concepts, approaches, or methods? Are the aims original and innovative? Does the project challenge existing paradigms or develop new methodologies or technologies?

Investigator: Is the investigator appropriately trained and well suited to carry out this work? Is the work proposed appropriate to the experience, level of the PI and other researchers (if any)?

Environment: Does the scientific environment in which the work will be done contribute to the probability of success? Do the proposed experiments take advantage of unique features of the scientific environment or employ useful collaborative arrangements ? Is there evidence of organizational support?

Also, in accordance with NIH policy, study section members are required to review applications with respect to a) the adequacy of the investigator's plans to include both men and women, inclusion of minority groups, and recruitment and retention; b) the reasonableness of the proposed budget and length of the project; and c) adequacy of protection of human subjects or animals.

11.3 SCORES AND CATEGORIES OF ACCEPTANCE AND REJECTION

How are applications scored and what are the possible outcomes of a review? Categories of acceptance and rejection vary from agency to agency. Let's first consider the system used by the Public Health Service and then examine the Department of Education.

> *Public Health Service:* The PHS uses a scoring system such that the best possible score is 1.00 and the worst is 5.00 and each application is scored to two figures (1.50). Box 11-2 outlines the scoring system.

BOX 11-2

NIH SCORING SYSTEM

Outstanding	1.0–1.90
Excellent	2.0–3.0
Satisfactory	3.0–4.0
Fair	4.0–5.0
Marginally acceptable	5.0

Each application that is discussed by the study section is given one score that reflects the final overall appraisal of the review panel. The individual scores of each panel are averaged and multiplied by 100 to yield a single overall priority score (e.g., 150). At the study section meeting, reviewers are then asked to spread final scores of approved applications to achieve a median score of 300. Approved applications are those which the IRG evaluates as having, "significant and substantial scientific and technical merit."

For most competitions, the Institutes also compute a *percentile rank*. This percentile rank indicates the position of a priority score compared to all priority scores assigned by that IRG in its last three meetings. The calculation of the percentile rank includes all applications, even those that were not given a full review by the study section (e.g., those applications who initially scored too high). For example, a percentile rank of 20 means that only 20% of the applications reviewed by that study section during the last three meetings had equal or better priority scores. These two scores serve as the primary indices of scientific merit and are a major factor in determining whether an application is actually funded.

Some agencies for certain competitions also determine a *percentile pay line*, which is a score based primarily on availability of funds. In these agencies, applications that have a percentile rank equal to or better than the percentile pay line are funded. In other agencies, the proposal that has the highest percentile rank is funded first. Funding proceeds with the next highest ranked proposals until the available money runs out. For agencies that do not compute a percentile rank, the proposal with the highest priority score is funded first. Investigators who are funded from the initial pool of money are usually notified by a letter sent to the University single point of contact, usually the office of research administrator. Prior to this notification, some agencies will notify your local congressman about the funding. Investigators can also contact the program officer to inquire about the funding status of their proposal.

Approved proposals whose scores are not high enough for the first round of funding are placed on a waiting list arranged by percentile rank or priority score. Applications on this list may receive either full or partial funding if additional money becomes available. These proposals are eligible for funding for up to one year. Unfortunately, after the initial distribution of funds, future funding is rare for these approved proposals.

If the study section decides that an application does not demonstrate sufficient scientific or technical merit, it is placed in the *Not Recommended for Further Consideration (NRFC)* category. Proposals in this category tend to demonstrate conceptual, scientific, or technical weakness. That is, the project idea may not be is scientifically sound or adequately developed, it may not match the priorities of the agency, the methodology may be unsound or significantly flawed, or the design may be in conflict with the rights of human subjects. This action is serious and indicates that the application will not be considered in the future for funding in its current form. Although you may resubmit the proposal idea, it will need to be substantially changed before you do. You o will need to give careful consideration to the reviewers' comments, and discuss your proposed revisions with a project officer who can advice you whether the agency will accept a future submission.

In some cases, a study section may decide that they cannot make an accurate decision about an application until additional or supplemental information is obtained. How the information is obtained depends upon the nature of the competition and the information that is required. For simple issues which need clarification, such as a budget item, missing letter of support, consortium agreement, or institutional review board approval, a project officer will contact the investigator by telephone. Other substantive issues raised by a panel may need to be addressed in written form. For example, the review panel may request clarification or additional information regarding a particular aspect of the study design. If this is the case, you must prepare a written justification or revision to the original procedures and submit it to the project officer for final review and approval.

In some competitions, especially those involving the development of a large "center" for research or training, a site visit is performed. The site visit is performed by a representative from the funding agency and either all members of the review panel or just the primary and secondary reviewers. This site visit may last from one to three days depending upon the nature of the competition and the extent to which there is a need to clarify the proposed activities. During the site visit, all members of the proposed project team must be present and a formal agenda followed. The site visitors may question you on any aspect of the proposal and also examine the physical resources of your institution. Following the site visit, the reviewers will prepare an additional report and make a final recommendation for funding. This is evaluated by the project officer who may also make specific suggestions as to funding and whether a substantive change in budget or procedures are necessary.

Department of Education—Funding agencies within the Department of Education follow a different set of scoring procedures. For most competitions, a proposal is rated on a scale of 0-100 in which 100 represents the best possible score and 0 the worst, based on an from three to five reviewers. Each section of a proposal has a point value attached to it, unlike in the NIH review. The reviewers evaluate and assign points to each section independently and then have the opportunity to revise these scores based upon the group discussion. An overall score of the proposal is then calculated to represent the average of each panel member's total score. Approved proposals are those that receive a panel rating of 80 or above. However, for most competitions, a score of 90 or above is necessary to actually receive funding. Those that are scored below 80 are classified as disapproved.

The following is an example of how three reviewers might evaluate a proposal:

BOX 11-3

Section/Criterion	Point Value	Reviewers' Score		
		1	2	3
1. Evidence of Need	0-10	8	9	9
2. Relevance	0-10	8	8	8
3. Plan of Operation	0-30	25	26	19
4. Nature of Curriculum	0-20	18	19	12
5. Quality of Personnel	0-10	9	9	8
6. Budget/Cost-effectiveness	0-10	9	9	8
7. Evaluation Plan	0-5	5	5	4
8. Adequacy of Resources	0-5	5	5	5
Total	**100**	**87**	**90**	**73**

The agency project staff then meet to discuss the proposals in funding range and evaluate their fit with the agency's mission and long-term goals. For the most part, the agency funds the proposal that receives the highest panel rating and continues funding proposals in descending order of their rating (all above 80) until the money runs out. However, it is possible for a highly rated proposal to not be funded if another proposal more closely fits the agency's perspective. As you can see, the proposal in the example above received a total average score of 83. This score is just within the funding range, but since it is close to the cut off score of 80, it is unlikely that it would be funded in this round. If you examine the pattern of scores, you will see that there was a significant discrepancy among the reviewers. Two of the reviewers scored the proposal much higher than the third reviewer. To resubmit the application, it would be important to first understand the areas of disagreement among the reviewers, obtain feedback from the program officer, and clearly address the issues raised by the third reviewer.

The Bureau of Health Professions uses a third method of scoring proposals. The Bureau uses the same scoring design as the Department of Education, with 100 being the best possible score and 0 being the worst. However, there are three differences in the way funding decisions are made: 1) they do not usually publish the point values for each section of the proposal; 2) they determine approved and disapproved proposals based on the review panel's recommendation, before scores are assigned; and 3) they rank the average score of approved proposals from high to low and continue funding until funds are depleted.

11.4 RESUBMISSION OPTIONS

The reason for non-funding may differ for each agency, competition, and proposal. Resubmitting a rejected proposal is part of the process of grantsmanship and is a reality for even the most experienced grant writer. Although no one likes a rejection, even the most skilled grant writer may not succeed in securing an award on the first submission of an application. You may need to submit an application up to three times prior to receiving an award. For agencies other than the NIH, you may even be allowed to submit more than three times. However, if you are not funded by the third attempt, you should carefully reevaluate your proposal idea, its competitiveness, and appropriateness for the agency to which you are submitting.

What are your options if you are not funded?—Keep in mind that in some competitions, such as those sponsored by certain foundations, or those for a contract or specific Request for Applications (RFA), there is not always the opportunity to resubmit a non-funded grant application. However, if it is permissible to resubmit an application, there are three steps in making a determination as to whether you should. These include analyzing:

- the priority score
- the reviewers' comments
- your discussions with a project officer

a. *Analyzing the priority score*—If your proposal was submitted to the PHS, you should carefully examine both the priority score and the percentile rank. Both scores provide an indication of the strength of your proposal. The priority score indicates its technical or scientific merit, whereas the percentile rank compares it to other proposals evaluated in the funding cycle. The percentile rank also provides an indication of how close you were to being funded.

For example, in the NIH system, a score of 2.5 to 3.5 implies that the proposal idea has merit but perhaps the design lacked sufficient detail. Scores in the range of 4.0to 5.0 suggest that the reviewers may not have liked the proposal idea or the design may have had serious flaws. In the latter case, major revisions are necessary before resubmitting to the next funding cycle.

Let's say you receive a score of 210 and a percentile rank of 20%. If the agency funds up to 18%, then you know you were very close to being funded.

If you submitted an application to the Department of Education, you need to assess both your overall score and the score from each reviewer. In the previous example, the proposal received a total average score of 83 but was not funded. Since a score of "80" is the cut-off point for eligibility of funding, you know you were very close. Had all three scores of the reviewers been close to 80, it would have indicated that the panel was consistent as to how they judged the quality of your proposal although they might not have been very excited about the idea or the methodology. But the opposite may also be tree. In the case above, the two high scores indicate that your proposal has funding potential but that at least one reviewer had significant concerns.

Usually, proposals with scores less than 60 indicate that the panel found significant problems that you need to address. If these issues can be addressed, then a resubmission may be warranted. However, if the panel expresses disinterest in the topic area, a fatal flaw in the design, or a substantial issue that you cannot address, then you probably should not resubmit the proposal.

b. *Reading and interpreting reviewers' comments*—After receiving an official letter or telephone call informing you about the funding decision, you will obtain a copy of the reviewers' comments (the "pink sheets"). The format of the summary sheet varies from agency to agency. Some agencies provide an overall evaluation of your proposal and separate scores, as well as evaluative comments that are made by each panel member. Other agencies provide a summary of the major strengths and weaknesses that were identified during the panel discussion. Still others will just list the major strengths and weaknesses. The pink sheets from NIH typically contain the following information:

1) A comprehensive description of your project and the proposed methodology

2) This is followed by a one to three page critique of each section of the proposal with particular emphasis on method

3) Then, the adequacy of each of the five criteria listed above is described, including publishing record and expertise to carry out the project

4) There is a brief appraisal of the adequacy of the proposed budget and concerns about human subjects

5) It concludes with a summary statement as to the recommendation for funding

Regardless of the form, the comments by a review panel should be carefully evaluated because they identify the issues that will need to be addressed in the resubmission of the proposal.

Take a deep breath before reading comments of the review panel. New investigators, as well as those who have received many awards, find it difficult to accept criticism found in the review. Some comments will be straightforward and identify a particular weakness. For example, "There is no budget justification." Other comments may be less direct and open to multiple interpretations. Let's say you received the following comment:

"While this appears to be an intriguing intervention, it is difficult to see how the results will have a significant impact on the day-to-day behavior of practicing therapists."

One interpretation of this comment is that the reviewers liked the idea, but did not think its significance was clearly communicated. The second interpretation is that the reviewers did not think the intervention would make a significant impact. If the first interpretation were correct, you would need to carefully explain the significance of the intervention for practice in a resubmission. If the second interpretation is correct, then you would need to reexamine the intervention and decide whether it is as significant as you believe. Sometimes it is difficult to discern which interpretation is accurate. In this case, discussing the critique with the project officer and sharing the intervention with colleagues to elicit feedback will assist you in determining the best approach in a resubmission.

As you read and interpret the pink sheets, look for comments that say "yes" and comments that say "no" for a resubmission. Consider the examples that are in Box 11-4. Panel members often try to encourage investigators, particularly for proposals that present innovative, interesting ideas but may not be fully developed and ready for funding. On rare occasions, review panels will encourage resubmission of proposals that are disapproved. This usually occurs when the proposal contains a highly innovative or important idea, but which may not have been fully developed. On the other hand, they may also send the opposite message if they do not think the proposal will be competitive even if it is revised.

Finally, some proposals contain what are called "fatal flaws." A fatal flaw represents a fundamental problem with the design or proposed program that cannot be remedied. A fatal flaw requires you to rethink the entire project idea and set of procedures. Box 11-5 provides an example.

BOX 11-4

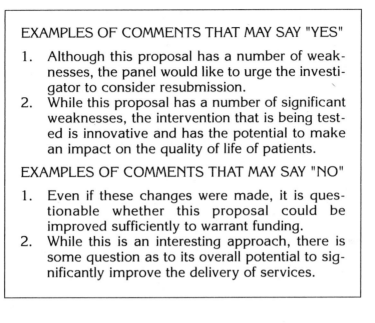

EXAMPLES OF COMMENTS THAT MAY SAY "YES"

1. Although this proposal has a number of weaknesses, the panel would like to urge the investigator to consider resubmission.
2. While this proposal has a number of significant weaknesses, the intervention that is being tested is innovative and has the potential to make an impact on the quality of life of patients.

EXAMPLES OF COMMENTS THAT MAY SAY "NO"

1. Even if these changes were made, it is questionable whether this proposal could be improved sufficiently to warrant funding.
2. While this is an interesting approach, there is some question as to its overall potential to significantly improve the delivery of services.

BOX 11-5

COMMENTS THAT ILLUSTRATE A FATAL FLAW

It is apparent that this intervention would require a minimum involvement of between eight and ten hours per day of clinical staff time, which does not appear feasible given the staffing levels of the participating clinical sites.

This research design cannot be accomplished without random assignment of patients to experimental and control groups. It does not appear that this is possible since to do so would compromise patient treatment plans at this facility. Without random assignment, however, it is difficult to see how the study outcomes can be interpreted.

Comments from a review panel can guide you in making a decision as to whether to resubmit and the kinds of changes that would be necessary to improve the proposal. You may want to share the comments or pink sheets with colleagues to obtain their reading of the panel's deliberations. Box 11-6 provides a strategy you may choose to follow for reviewing pink sheets or summary statements from the review.

BOX 11-6

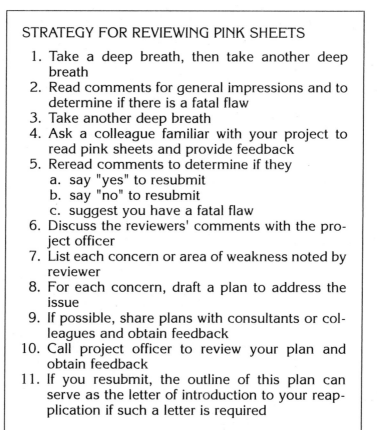

STRATEGY FOR REVIEWING PINK SHEETS

1. Take a deep breath, then take another deep breath
2. Read comments for general impressions and to determine if there is a fatal flaw
3. Take another deep breath
4. Ask a colleague familiar with your project to read pink sheets and provide feedback
5. Reread comments to determine if they
   a. say "yes" to resubmit
   b. say "no" to resubmit
   c. suggest you have a fatal flaw
6. Discuss the reviewers' comments with the project officer
7. List each concern or area of weakness noted by reviewer
8. For each concern, draft a plan to address the issue
9. If possible, share plans with consultants or colleagues and obtain feedback
10. Call project officer to review your plan and obtain feedback
11. If you resubmit, the outline of this plan can serve as the letter of introduction to your reapplication if such a letter is required

c. *Discussions with project officers*—It is very important to talk to the program officer who was involved with the review panel or, in the NIH, the Scientific Review Administrator. He or she may have insights as to the discussion that occurred among panelists. Program officers are adept at interpreting reviewers written comments and they may be able to provide specific suggestions to improve your proposal based on these comments. A program officer may not encourage you to resubmit if your idea does not fit agency priorities or the review panel had substantive issues with the project. If your program officer did not attend the panel discussion, he or she may encourage you to discuss specific questions about the review with the SRA in the case of the NIH or the project officer who did sit on the study section.

In addition to discussing the nature of the review panel's deliberation and their comments, other questions may help you understand where your application is placed in relation to the others that were submitted. Examples of questions you may want to pose to a program officer are listed in Box 11-7.

BOX 11-7

WHAT TO ASK A PROGRAM OFFICER ABOUT THE REVIEW

1. How many applications were submitted?
2. How many grants were funded?
3. What were the priority scores of funded grants?
4. Given reviewer comments and score, would resubmission be recommended?
5. Will the same panel of reviewers evaluate a resubmission?
6. How should you indicate that the application is a resubmission?

d. *Considerations in a resubmission*—Let's say you finally receive notification from the agency that your proposal was approved but not funded. Your priority score was reasonably high, the review panel did not cite any major weaknesses on the pink sheets, and the program officer confirms the panel's enthusiasm. If she encourages you to revise the proposal for the next funding cycle, you should meet with your project team to determine if resubmission is feasible. If you and your team decide revisions, here are some points to consider when resubmitting:

1. Remember that a resubmission needs to be given the same careful thought as the original proposal. Do not assume that only a few editorial changes based on the suggestions of the review panel will suffice. One effective strategy is to put the panel suggestions in one of three categories: major changes, minor changes, and editorial changes. Major changes are those that require you to change a substantive part of the proposal. An example of a major change in an educational grant may be a modification in the sequence or content of the courses, modification in objectives and evaluation procedures, or addition or readjustment of the overall program. In a research grant, an example of a major change is a revision in the design, analytic direction, or instrument.

   Minor changes are those that require additional information that augments the proposal or statements that clarify procedures. For example, if you did not include adequate information in your statement of need for the project or a clear plan for self-sufficiency, you would need to gather additional information to include in these sections.

   Editorial changes are those that require you to rewrite portions of a section to assure greater clarity, to correct typographical errors, or to add figures or tables that summarize and clarify major points. Start working on the major changes first, since they will require the most effort and time.

2. Most agencies require that you indicate the application represents a resubmission. Ask the program officer how best to present this to the review panel. Each

agency has a different set of requirements for the way in which to provide such notification. For most applications you may need to highlight the substantive narrative changes you make by either bolding the section or neatly drawing a vertical line in the margin by the section. Let the reviewers know in your summary page or cover letter how you have demarcated the major revisions. Some agencies require a cover letter while others request that a one-page summary be included in the body of the narrative. In either case, you need to indicate that you carefully reviewed the recommendations by the panel and have revised and strengthened your proposal in accordance to their comments. Also, briefly outline the major changes that you have made.

3. Remember that you need to update all materials, including literature reviews, biographical information, funding information and letters of support.

4. Depending upon your interpretation of the first review you received, you may want to request that an individual with special expertise be assigned to review the resubmission. For example, let's say you proposed an ethnographic study and the panel members only had expertise in quantitative designs. You may request that an anthropologist be appointed to the review panel so that there is representation of the expertise that is required to review your application.

If you believe that you received an unfair review, you do have some recourse. You can submit a letter of complaint to your program officer or the branch chief of the agency. We should stress that this option should be used only for a glaring injustice and not because you disagree with the panel's decision. The only reason for you to write a letter like this would be to help improve the review system. You will not receive a reversal in your score or funding. For more information concerning NIH's peer review process, go to the following Web site: http://www.csr.nih.gov and http://www.csr.nih.gov/review/policy.asp. Information also is available by e-mail at DDER@nih.gov or GrantsInfo@nih.gov, or by calling, writing, or faxing a request to CSR. For more information about the

Department of Education's peer review approaches search their web site for the competition of relevance. Go to http://www.ed.gov/search or http://www.ed.gov/pubs/peerreview/execsumm.html.

SUMMARY

Five major points have been made in describing the proposal review process, categories of acceptance and rejection, your options for resubmitting a non-funded project, and your responsibilities in the post-award phase.

1. The review process is an arduous and time-consuming activity in which proposals are given a fair and thorough review. It is very important to present a clearly written proposal . that closely follows the proposal outline prepared by the agency to help facilitate the review process and improve your chances of funding.

2. Two major federal funding sources for health and human service projects, the Department of Education and the Public Health Service, have different systems for evaluating proposals. Understanding these systems will help you determine the appropriateness of resubmitting your proposal if it is not funded the first time.

3. The majority of proposals submitted to a competition are approved, but not funded. This tends to reflect the lack of money available to federal agencies, rather than the quality of the projects that are submitted. Therefore, it is important for you to learn and avoid the common mistakes in non-funded proposals so that you can improve your chances of funding.

4. If you are not funded upon your first submission, which is common, there are three ways to determine whether you should resubmit a revised application. These are an analysis of the priority score, an analysis of the reviewers' comments, and discussions with a program officer.

5. Review panels communicate explicitly and implicitly important suggestions to applicants. Therefore, it is critical to read the reviewers' comments carefully and pay close attention to their comments.

Key Acronyms Related to the Review Process

CSR—Center for Scientific Review
DRG—Division of Research Grants—now referred to as CSR
GAN—Grant Award Notice from the Department of Education
IRG—Integrated Research Group
SRA—Scientific Review Administrator
NIH—National Institutes of Health
NGA—Notice of Grant Award from the NIH
PHS—Public Health Service
ORA—Office of Research Administration

Chapter 12

A Case Study

- Excerpt From a Proposal
- A Critique

Remember Ms. L. from chapter 1? She was interested in developing an educational program to prepare an interdisciplinary group of students to work with residents of homeless shelters. Let's see what has happened to Ms. L. and her team.

If you recall, she had been advised to cast a wide net to identify external funding sources and develop a team involving other health and human service professionals. After searching for funding agencies using the sources described in chapter 2, she and her team identified 10 foundations from the *Foundation Directory* and obtained a computer listing of federal agencies about an inch thick from an electronic search conducted by the reference librarian. These searches generated a number of agencies that appeared interested in funding a range of programs for underserved populations. The team then began to review the information about each of the agencies to determine whether there was a potential match between each agency's funding priorities and the original idea of the project. After reviewing descriptions of the foundations, the team concluded that their idea did not match any of the priorities identified. They then spent the next few weeks examining the web sites of federal agencies that sponsor likely programs. They reviewed the goals and funding priorities of each, titles of previously funded projects, size of awards, and due dates for the next competition. They also identified the program officers in charge of each competition.

From this review the team identified four potential funding sources whose priorities seemed relevant to their idea. They spent the next two months refining their ideas, updating their literature review and developing a two-page concept paper describing their proposed project.

Ms. L. then called the program officers in each of the agencies they had identified from the web site. She introduced herself to the program officers and explained her team's idea and asked if she could make an appointment to visit the agency in the next month. She also asked if they would be willing to review their concept paper for discussion at the meeting. Two of the program officers agreed and a date was set for the meeting. The third program officer apologized, indicating that his agency would be in the midst of reviewing proposals on the planned date and that he would not be available. He did agree to review the concept paper and suggested that Ms. L. schedule a conference call in about two weeks, so he could discuss the project with the team. The fourth program officer also apologized, saying that she would be conducting site visits of some of her funded projects during Ms. L.'s planned visit, but that she planned to attend the annual meeting of Ms. L.'s professional association which was scheduled for the following week. The program officer agreed to review the concept paper and meet with Ms. L. during the conference.

At the professional meeting, Ms. L. and the program officer met during one of the coffee breaks between sessions to discuss the concept paper. The program officer indicated that she liked the idea of the project and thought that it had potential for funding, but felt that the proposed budget was a little higher than her agency normally funded. She also suggested that the closing date for the agency's next competition was too close for Ms. L. and her team to put together a competitive proposal, even if they were able to reduce the budget. Finally, she suggested another agency that would have interest in the project idea. Ms. L. was heartened by the last remark, since the suggested agency was one they had identified.

When Ms. L. returned to her university, it was time for the scheduled conference call to the next funding agency. During the call, the program officer encouraged the team to pursue their idea, and gave them a number of suggestions to make the project stronger. However, he told them that the primary focus of his agency was on homeless women and children. He asked them if it would be possible for them to change the focus of their project to this population. Ms. L. thanked him for his suggestions and indicated that they would seriously think about the change of focus.

After the call, the team discussed the possibility of revising their idea, but decided that their real interest lay in helping the homeless men, who made up the bulk of the residents of the shelters they were working in.

A week later, Ms. L. made the trip to Washington and visited the last two of the agencies they had identified. She found both of the program officers to be very friendly and helpful. At the first agency the program officer told her that, while he thought the team's idea was a good one, his agency was really more interested in rural, underserved populations. He did, however, provide some suggestions about how to strengthen the team's project. Ms. L.'s second meeting was much more encouraging. Dr. C., the program officer, indicated that her agency was very interested in programs providing services to medically underserved communities. She also said that her agency strongly encouraged both interdisciplinary approaches and demonstrated linkages between universities and community agencies. Dr. C. then made some suggestions for improving the teams' proposed plan and identified an announcement in the *Federal Register* and on the agency web site. An excerpt of this announcement is shown in Box 12-1.

BOX 12-1

EXCERPT OF AN ANNOUNCEMENT

Section 767 authorizes the Secretary to award grants to eligible entities to assist such entities in meeting the costs associated with expanding or establishing programs that will increase the number of individuals trained in allied health professions. Programs funded under this section may include:

1. those that establish community-based training programs that link academic centers to medically underserved or rural communities in order to increase the number of individuals trained;
2. those that expand or establish demonstration centers to emphasize innovative models to link allied health clinical practice, education, and research;

BOX 12-1 *(Continued)*

3. those that establish interdisciplinary training programs that promote the effectiveness of allied health practitioners in the areas of prevention and health promotion, geriatrics, long-term care, ethics, and rehabilitation.

    To maximize program benefit, programs that provide financial assistance in the form of traineeships to students will not be considered for funding.

When preparing the detailed description of the Innovative Project Grant, information should be presented according to the following outline:

I.   Background and Rationale
II.   Objectives
III. Project Methods
IV.   Evaluation
V.   Applicant Summary and Resources
VI.   Budget and Justification
VII. Self-Sufficiency

Special Consideration

In determining the order of funding of approved applications, special consideration will be given to the following:

Applicants demonstrating affiliation agreements for interdisciplinary training experiences in nursing homes, hospitals, or community centers for underserved populations.

Applicants demonstrating affiliation agreements with migrant health facilities.

Funding

Approximately $1,900,000 will be available in the current fiscal year for this program. It is anticipated that approximately 10 new awards will be made, with a period of support not to exceed three years.

Excited, Ms. L. returned to her university and shared the announcement and feedback with members of her team, who decided to submit an application to this competition and request special consideration. As a first step in proposal development, Ms. L. and her team identified the roles each would assume to write the proposal (as described in chapter 8) and on the project itself, if it was funded.

The following section presents excerpts from the team's proposal, which is then followed by its critique.

12.1 EXCERPT FROM A PROPOSAL

Title: *A Program to Train Interdisciplinary Health Care Teams to Work With the Homeless*

   I.   Background and Rationale

     Introduction and Purpose of the Project

The departments of social work, occupational therapy, physical therapy, and nursing at the University of Excalibar, propose to develop, implement and evaluate a new program by which to educate students to provide interdisciplinary community-based health care including health promotion and restorative services to individuals who are homeless.

This three-year project will be accomplished in three overlapping phases: development, implementation, and evaluation. The development phase involves the formation of a partnership among social work, allied health, and nursing faculty and community leaders. The purpose of this partnership is to plan and implement a new program of didactic and clinical experiences for students in each of the programs. The implementation phase involves executing the collaboratively derived educational activities. Didactic and experiential community-based interdisciplinary training opportunities will be designed to move the student from an independent practitioner with a unidisciplinary focus to a collaborator and member of an interdisciplinary, community-based team. The evaluation phase involves appraising the success of the project. Evaluation will be conducted by the Community Advisory Board, which will assess the effectiveness of the program.

Changing Needs and Growing Numbers of Homeless

This project targets the homeless because of the demonstrated lack of health care services for this population, their clear need for both comprehensive health promotion and health restoration services, and the cost-effective role of nursing and allied health professionals in the delivery of such services. As a heterogeneous group with complex and diverse health care needs, this population challenges the present service delivery system and underscores the pressing need for community-based strategies that are effective, culturally appropriate, and comprehensive.

Who Are The Homeless?

Homelessness is defined as an individual who "lacks a fixed, regular, and adequate night-time residence; or has a primary night time residency that is 1) a supervised publicly or privately operated shelter designed to provide temporary living accommodations; or 2) an institution that provides a temporary residence for individuals intended to be institutionalized. Since the 1980's, homelessness has increased in the United States due, in part , to a decreased availability of affordable housing. Those who are most affected are individuals who are poor with limited education and job skills; those who have mental illness and substance abuse issues; and women and children affected by domestic violence. It is estimated that 6.5% of individuals in the United States have been homeless at some point in their life, and 3.6% of individuals had been homeless sometime between 1989 and 1994. Based on existing demographic data, there is consensus that the current homeless population ranges in age between 35–40 on average. At least one-half of the population is non-white. Thus, national statistics strongly support the need for the model program that is proposed in this application.

II. Goals and Objectives

The primary goal of the proposed program is to test an approach for developing a new community-based health care program in education, service, and research for an underserved population.

There are three specific program objectives to accomplish this goal.

Objective #1: Participate in year-long activities to develop a curriculum.

Objective #2: Expand the knowledge base and clinical abilities of faculty and community-based providers for the homeless so that they can develop and teach an innovative interdisciplinary curriculum focused on community-based health care for the homeless population.

Objective #3: Enable faculty, in collaboration with community-based providers for the homeless, to understand and apply the linkages among theory-based practice, research, and policy formation to curriculum development.

III. Project Methods

The specific activities in each project phase are based upon a proven learning process to develop competence in interdisciplinary team approaches. This process first involves faculty and student mastery of discipline-specific knowledge and skills in clinical decision making, clinical leadership, and health care delivery systems. Building upon "uni-disciplinary" knowledge and skill, participants will explore potential multidisciplinary relationships. Finally, through specially designed course work in team building and practicum experiences in community-based team care, faculty and students will gain competence in working on interdisciplinary, community-based teams.

IV. Evaluation

The evaluation process will determine the extent to which the program represents an effective and workable model for preparing social work, physical therapy, occupational therapy, and nursing students to work on interdisciplinary community-based teams. To this end, the Project Director will charge the Community Advisory Board with overseeing and guiding the systematic evaluation of each phase and component of the program with special emphasis on assessing the training curriculum. Both a formative and summative evaluation process will be developed.

V. Budget and Justification

Project Director (Ms. L.): Ms. L. will devote 35% of her time to the project. She will direct the didactic and clinical curriculum development activities and serve as liaison to participating social service agencies and community advocates for the homeless. She will also work with each department representative to coordinate the clinical activities of each department.

Department Representatives (Dr. G., Ms. L., Dr. T.): These individuals will each devote a 10% effort and will be involved in curriculum planning, teach a specially designed course in the program, recruit and advise students from each of their departments, and serve as advisors to student research projects.

Supplies:

Clerical supplies, postage, telephone, and minor occupational and physical therapy equipment, such as splinting material and foam theraband, will be required to support the operation of the project. An amount of $3,500 during each year of the project is requested.

Staff Travel:

Travel funds in the amount of $5,200 for the first year, $5,000 during the second year, and $6,000 in the third year is being requested. Funds will be used for local travel by faculty, travel to three professional conferences, and travel to an international meeting in London, England, on homelessness.

Trainee Expenses:

Partial support for the 16 students in the program is requested. A stipend of $2,000/student/year is requested.

Appendices

A: Letter of support from a community shelter

B: Curriculum vitae of project personnel

C: Selected publications of project team

12.2 A CRITIQUE

The teams' proposal arrived at the Grants Management Office of the Bureau of Health Professions on the day of the deadline. It was logged in and assigned a unique identification number. One hundred and twenty proposals were received for the competition and the program officer was very busy organizing three, 10-person review panels. Each reviewer received eight proposals, four to review as a primary reviewer and four to review as a secondary reviewer. The proposals were mailed to the reviewers six weeks before the scheduled panel meeting.

Ms. L.'s proposal was reviewed on the second day of deliberations. Although the proposal was well written and avoided the common writing problems identified in chapter 8, there were some fundamental issues raised by the review panel. Can you identify the issues reviewers might have had? Here is an outline of some of the strengths and weaknesses of the proposal that would have been raised by a review panel.

Strengths:

1. This is a well-written, innovative approach that appears to have the potential to improve the health status of an underserved population.

2. National data on the homeless population and a strong justification for the need for services for this population is provided.

3. The proposal addresses a critical need for training students to work with an underserved population.

4. The involvement of multiple disciplines and the emphasis of the program on both health promotion and restoration is an important approach to solving the complex problems facing individuals who are homeless.

5. The organization of three project phases represents a logical ordering of activities to accomplish the two goals of the project.

6. The involvement of members of the community and academic faculty in the implementation of this project appears to have the potential for ensuring it's success.

7. The project director has had extensive experience working within shelters for the homeless and organizing a volunteer program for students.

8. The project team seems well qualified to conduct this project

Weaknesses:

1. Although the national significance of developing a program to serve the homeless is adequately demonstrated, the applicant does not provide sufficient data or information as to the local need for and benefit of this program. It is unclear whether there are any such programs existing in the applicant's region and no needs assessment is presented.

2. The applicant proposes to develop curriculum materials based on a partnership and collaboration between community members and academic faculty. However, there is insufficient evidence of the involvement of key community members and an inadequate plan for the development of such a collaborative relationship. Such a partnership should involve members of the community in the actual planning of the grant.

3. There is only one letter of support from one of the shelters that will be involved in the program. Support letters from the other shelters and key members of the community would be advisable to assure that this is a feasible program and acceptable to the shelters.

4. The plan for evaluation is weak and underdeveloped. Although the use of a Community Advisory Board to assist in the evaluation is appropriate, there is no specification as to how they are going to evaluate the program, the criteria which will be used, or the process by which the evaluation will be carried out.

5. Objective #1 is stated as an activity so it is difficult to determine what will be accomplished or who will participate in the curriculum development activities.

6. There is no strong reason given for why the professions that will participate in the program were chosen, what important health need they will provide, or what evidence exists that they will be cost effective. Absent from the multidisciplinary group are nutritionists, dental hygienists, educators, job placement counselors, and others who have important skills to contribute to the care and well-being of the homeless.

7. It is unclear as to the ultimate goal of this project—is it the provision of service to the homeless or development of an education program for students in the health professions?

8. Although the budget appears appropriate to accomplish the activities of the program, the applicant requests funds for trainee expenses. This expense is disallowed in this competition.

9. Applicant also requests funds for travel to an international meeting. Government funds can not be used for travel outside of the United States except to Canada and Mexico.

Based on this review, the panel approved the proposal but assigned it a score of 65 out of a possible 100 (see chapter 11 for a discussion of scoring procedures). When Ms. L. contacted Dr. C., the project officer in the Bureau to discuss their score, she was told that it was probably just outside the range for funding. However, Dr. C. also told her that the review panel was sending a clear and positive message to her and her team. This message was that the program was innovative and of great importance, but needed further refinement, particularly in the plan for implementation and evaluation. Look again at each weakness that was identified. Each point can easily be addressed by Ms. L. and her team. The review panel did not identify a fatal flaw.

Although very disappointed with their score, Ms. L. and her team decided to resubmit the application. Let's review how they used the reviewers' comments as a guide to develop their resubmission.

There were 9 weaknesses cited by the review panel. The first had to do with the lack of data on local need for the program, the existence of other programs in the region, and the lack of a needs assessment. Ms. L. assigned one of her team members to update the literature review of the original proposal and to conduct a new review of local statistics on the homeless population. Other members of the team conducted a needs assessment. They met with representatives of city and county social services agencies to determine what programs were available to individuals who were homeless and to identify the most pressing physical, mental, medical, and social needs of this population.

The second weakness suggested that there was no community input into the planning of the proposed curriculum materials or in the grant project itself. In conducting the needs assessment, members of the team had made contact with a number of community leaders. The team decided to expand the size of their Community Advisory Board by asking some of these individuals to participate. At the first meeting of the Board, Ms. L. divided the members into three small task groups. She asked one of the groups to review the curriculum materials and a second to review the overall project plan of action and make suggestions for improvement. The third task group was asked to develop an evaluation plan for the project, which was the fourth weakness identified by the review panel. Once these tasks were completed, the team began revising the application.

The first step was to incorporate the results of the updated and expanded literature review and needs assessment into the introduction and rational section of the proposal, and add a paragraph explaining the rationale for the selection of the four professions to participate in the project (weaknesses #1 and #6). They then clarified the goal of the project (weakness #7), by indicating that the primary goal was to develop a program to prepare interdisciplinary groups of students to provide health care services to individuals residing in four homeless shelters. Following this, objective #1 was rewritten as: "Develop curriculum materials to enable students to work as members of an interdisciplinary team in the provision of health care services to individuals who are homeless" (weakness #5).

The team then made modifications to the section on project methods by clarifying the role of the Community Advisory Board, indicating that the Board would work collaboratively during the first year of the project to develop the interdisciplinary curriculum materials as specified in objective #1 (weakness #2).

In the evaluation section of the revised proposal, the team described the evaluation materials and the process by which they were developed by the task group of the Advisory Board. These materials were included in one of the appendices of the proposal (weakness #4).

The team then amended the budget by removing the requests for international travel and for traineeship money (weaknesses #8 and #9). Finally, they requested letters of support from community leaders on the Advisory Board, the heads of some of the major social services agencies in the city, and Directors of each of the participating shelters.

As you can see, addressing the weaknesses cited by the review panel was relatively time consuming, but not difficult. As part of the submission of the revised proposal, Ms. L. included a letter to the reviewers that outlined each weakness cited by the review panel and the teams' response. Upon completion of the revised proposal, Ms. L. and her team realized they had improved both their proposal and project significantly. The second review panel agreed, and funding was obtained on the second submission.

Part VI

Receiving the Grant Award

When you receive notification of an award (by letter, telephone, or sometimes by e-mail)—celebrate! A funded grant is a significant accomplishment and indicates that your proposal has been ranked very high in comparison to the other proposals submitted by your peers to that competition. You are now entering what is referred to as the "post-award" phase of grantsmanship. The post award phase involves not only the implementation of your proposed project, but also the management of the award. In chapter 13, we describe the key considerations in managing your grant award.

Chapter 13

Managing the Grant Award

- Federal agency requirements
- Notification and implementation process
- Common agency reports
- Institutional rules
- Budget management
- Academic policies

The requirements for managing a grant project go beyond conducting the science or following the educational training steps you have outlined in your proposal. In carrying out a project, there are a myriad of important administrative details that must be attended to by your institution, the funding agency, and you as the principal investigator or project director. There is a hierarchy of rules and regulations that are set forth by the funding agency, in addition to the specifications found in the terms of the particular award. It is also necessary for all of your project-related activities to comply with state and local laws and ethical standards of professional and clinical conduct.

This chapter identifies key federal agency regulations associated with funded projects, the interim and final reports that you will have to submit to a funding agency, and the specific offices in most universities that provide oversight to the requirements of a granting agency. It also describes critical policies regarding conflict of interest and authorship that you need to be aware of, as well as suggestions for managing your budget. While the focus is on federal rules and regulations, private foundations follow similar policies. Regardless of the funding source, most agencies engage in some form of monitoring of the activities of grantees, and thus it is important to learn the oversight and reporting structure.

13.1 FEDERAL AGENCY REGULATIONS

Recent high profile cases of research misconduct and financial irregularities that have been reported as occurring in a few elite universities have raised significant concern in the scientific community and the federal government. Although these cases maybe the minority, their transgressions have been so egregious that, in response, federal agencies have begun to monitor grants with more scrutiny. A number of new regulations, including required mandatory training programs, have been initiated to prevent misconduct in science and rectify poor research practices. The importance of following these regulations is critical. Violations can have serious implications for you as the principal investigator and for your institution. Most of these regulations emanate from the Office of Management and Budget (OMB) of the federal government and are found in three documents called OMB Circulars.

There are other rules and regulations that you must follow in addition to the OMB Circulars. First, each funding agency sets forth specific guidelines for all of their programs. These rules must fall within the framework outlined in the OMB circulars, but may be specific to a particular program. Second, an award notice also provides a specification of the terms of the award. For example, in the Department of Health and Human Services, most investigator-initiated grants are considered under "expanded authority" which allows the principal investigator to shift monies from one budget category to another (e.g., you can shift $500 from your supply line to your travel line), without notifying the agency. However, other grants not under expanded authority require written notification and approval for any such modifications. The third set of rules that must be followed are the policies and procedures set forth by your institution with regard to hiring and oversight of grant personnel, budgetary reporting, and Institutional Review Board requirements.

Box 13.1 contains a brief description and the web address where the OMB Circulars can be found along with the policy statements of the National Institutes of Health and the National Science Foundation. These references contain most of the regulations you need to know to manage your grant project. It is important to become familiar with the basic rules within each of these documents.

BOX 13.1

IMPORTANT RESOURCES IN GRANTS MANAGEMENT

OMB Circular A-21 is the federal "rule book" for university financial arrangements. It sets the rules for spending the money you receive in your grant and identifies allowable and nonallowable expenses. (http://whitehouse.gov/omb/circulars/a021.html)

OMB Circular A-110 sets the administrative standards for grants and other agreements. It is designed to assure that grants are managed consistently among all federal agencies. (http://whitehouse.gov/omb/circulars/a110/a110.html)

OMB Circular A-133 specifies the rules for audits of compliance with federal regulations. (http:whitehouse.gov/omb/circulars/a133/a133.html)

NIH Grants Policy sets specific rules for all grant projects funded by the NIH. (http://grants.nih.gov/grants/policy/nihgps_2001/)

NSF Grants Policy Manual sets specific rules for all grant projects funded by the National Science Foundation. (http://www.nsf.gov/pubs/stis1995/nsf9526.txt)

In addition to the regulations discussed above, a program officer who is assigned to your award will also monitor your grant. The degree of monitoring will vary from one agency to another as well as across specific competitions within one agency. In some cases, monitoring may occur through regular telephone contact or a periodic post-award site visit. However, for most grant awards, you will be required to submit a yearly written progress report and that will be your only contact with an officer. Keep in mind, however, that you must always notify a program officer of any significant changes or substantial difficulties that occur. For example, if you are unable to recruit study participants or if you are significantly delayed in implementing a particular grant-related activity, you should alert your program officer and discuss potential modifications to the project and strategies.

Keep in mind that funding agencies need to demonstrate the productivity of its grantees and the impact of its funding programs. Therefore, you should share any manuscripts, manuals, and products that result from your grant with the funding agency. Any materials that you develop as part of the grant effort are legally that of the funding agency. Remember to always provide a footnote indicating that your manuscript or product was developed as a result of support by the agency.

13.2 NOTIFICATION AND IMPLEMENTATION PROCESS

As we have discussed in chapter 4, a research or training grant is awarded to you through your institution. Your institution is legally responsible for the conduct of your project and for compliance to OMB rules and regulations. However, you are also held accountable. Usually, you will first receive the official notification of funding from someone in your institution designated as the "single point of contact." The federal government has initiated the "single point of contact" with universities and other agencies for the purpose of streamlining communications with those that they have funded. This means that all grant notifications and other correspondence is sent directly to a central office for distribution to all the appropriate grantees in the institution. If you are at a major university, this number can be very large, and the sheer volume of correspondence can result in delays in processing award notifications and other announcements. Recently, the federal government has begun to send these notices electronically, which greatly facilitates the process. Even so, you should learn who at your institution is the single point of contact. It is also important for you to become aware of the dates of expected notification of awards and the deadline dates for required reports. Do not hesitate to contact your single point of contact if you believe something has been delayed.

Grant notification from the NIH is referred to as the Notice of Grant Award (NGA). Once you receive the NGA, you should carefully review its specifications and the budget amounts that are allocated per year. If you have any questions or identify inconsistencies, then you must notify your research administration as well as the grant management office of the funding agency. Once the university has received the NGA, the budget office, often called the Sponsored Program Accounting Office (SPAO), will set up a special account for the grant budget. In some cases you are permitted to allocate expenditures to a grant that were incurred 90 days prior to the official notification.

13.3 COMMON AGENCY REPORTS

All funding agencies, private or federal, require periodic and standard reports of your budget expenses and progress in implementing the proposed activities. Each agency has its own requirements, so it is important to read the pertinent instructions or communicate with your officer so you know what is expected in these reports.

When you have received federal funding, there are three reports you must make for each year of the grant award: a progress report on your project; a budget reconciliation report; and an effort report. Whereas the progress and budget reports occur annually, effort reports are submitted periodically, usually every six months. Effort reports certify the amount of time each individual has worked on your grant.

Progress reports

Most multi-year grant projects are referred to as noncompeting renewals. Progress reports are required for each project year and funding for the next year is contingent on submitting a satisfactory progress report. The funding agency usually provides a detailed set of directions to write this report. For most NIH progress reports, the PHS 2590 forms must be used. Some agencies also require supplementary reports mandated by Congress. For example, the Bureau of Health Professions in the Department of Health and Human Services requires that you include a report on the number of minorities participating in your grant, either as trainees, research subjects, or faculty.

A few projects fall into a category called competing renewals. In this case, you need to prepare a much more detailed and persuasive progress report, since a panel will review your report in much the same way as your original application. It is best to confirm with your project officer the category your grant falls under.

Budget Reports

Each year you also have to make a report that summarizes your use of the funds allocated in the budget. Usually this report is compiled by the SPAO. However, you should maintain on-going communication with this office because you may have to provide them with information required for the report. You will also have to notify them of any changes to the budget. This SPAO will also compile the final budget report to the granting agency. Although you do not have to compile these reports, you will have to attest to their accuracy and sign the report. That is why it is essential that you maintain your own records of your grant expenses and carefully review the accounting records to assure that there are no discrepancies between your figures and the official reports. Both the yearly and final budget reports are due to the Office of Grants Management 90 days after the conclusion of the yearly grant cycle or the grant itself.

Effort Reporting

The federal government also requires all of their grantees to submit what are called effort reports. This report requires you, as the principal investigator or project director, to assure that each individual has devoted the required amount of time on the project over the past six months or year. For example, if you hired a statistician at 10% effort, you will need to certify that the individual actually spent that amount of time working on the project. If the individual worked more or less time, then you must alter the effort report to reflect the actual amount of time he or she worked on the grant. It is important to remember in completing this form that the amount of time or effort spent on a particular grant may not reflect the original budget that was allocated for that person. For example, a person may spend a 25% effort on a grant when only 10% of his or her time is actually paid for by the grant budget. Both of these categories will be reflected in the report. Effort reports are usually prepared by the Office of Research Administration or, in some institutions, an office of internal audit and sent to you periodically, usually every six months.

Final report

At the completion of your grant project, most agencies require that you submit a final report that summarizes your work effort and how you completed the project goals and objectives. There are usually standard forms or explicit directions for compiling this report. In the final report, you need to list any products, manuscripts in progress and press, and completed publications that were developed from the grant activity.

Carry-over funds

In a move toward efficiency, the federal government has initiated a policy referred to as Expanded Authorities. This is a mechanism in many grant programs that allows institutions and principal investigators some latitude in making budgetary decisions without the need for prior approval by the funding agency. Most federal grant programs fall under Expanded Authorities. If your grant is in this category, it will usually be noted in the Notice of Grant Award. Lately, however, the practice has become so common that many agencies now only indicate if your grant is an exception to the rule. If you have any question about this, talk to your Program Officer or to your ORA.

As part of the Expanded Authority, you are permitted to carry funds forward from one year to the next. That is, if by the end of a project year you have not spent all of the money authorized for that year, you are allowed to move a certain amount of the excess to the next project year without obtaining prior permission from the federal government. Under expanded authorities, you are allowed to carry forward 25% of the amount allotted for the current year without permission. To carry forward more than that amount, you need to obtain written approval from the agency. This will involve a letter from you explaining the reasons why all of the budgeted money was not spent and what you plan to use it for in the next year. Box 13.2 provides an example of how this might work.

BOX 13.2

AN EXAMPLE

Let's assume that Ms. L. had a first year budget for her training program of $100,000. She had antici-pated using $30,000 of this money to hire instruc-tors for the educational portion of the program. However, during the year she had trouble recruiting enough students to participate in the program and decided to offer it in year 2 instead. Under expand-ed authority she would be allowed to keep the $25,000 and add it to her year 2 budget.

Any amount of unspent money over 25% must be returned to the federal government if you can not present a compelling reason for why it was not spent that project year.

No cost extensions

If at the end of the final year of your grant, you have unspent money, it is possible to extend your grant and use this money to complete the grant activities. This is called a no-cost extension, since it is at no cost to the federal government. These extensions are usually granted for up to one year. Applying for an extension requires that you write a letter to the Grants Management Office in the funding agency at least 30 days prior to the end date of the grant. This letter should state the reasons for the request, the amount of money that you anticipate having left over, the amount of time you are requesting, and the activities you will undertake during the extension period.

BOX 13.3

AN EXAMPLE

Ms. L. is approaching the end of her grant funding and realizes that she still has $10,000 that she will not be able to spend. This money was originally designated to conduct an evaluation of the training program. Because the recruitment problems necessitated a delay in implementing the program, Ms. L. did not have adequate time to conduct the final evaluation. Ms. L. composed a letter to the Grants Management Office explaining the delay in program implementation caused by difficulties in recruitment and requested a six month no-cost extension to conduct the program evaluation.

13.4 INSTITUTIONAL RULES

In chapter 4 we discussed the importance of learning about the requirements of your institution prior to submitting a grant application. It is likewise important to understand the functions of the various offices at your institution that manage the post-award phase and oversee the regulations. Individuals in these offices will have an in-depth understanding of the OMB Circulars and will be able to help you through the morass of requirements. Box 13.4 contains a list of common grant administration offices with a description of their general responsibilities. In some institutions, these functions may be combined or referred to differently.

BOX 13.4

COMMON GRANTS ADMINISTRATION OFFICES

Office of Research Administration

- Single point of contact with the government for award notices and other correspondence
- Final signatory for all grants and contracts
- Negotiates indirect cost recovery rate for the institution
- Provides effort reports to the government
- Interprets the various rules and regulations that you have to follow

Office of Scientific Affairs

- Oversees animal and human subjects protection
- Oversees the Institutional Review Board
- Monitors institutional requirements for bio-safety
- Oversees clinical trials and establishes a Data Safety and Monitoring Board
- Maintains conflict of interest policy
- Investigates possible cases of misconduct in science
- Develops university research policies

Institutional Review Board

- Reviews and approves all protocols dealing with animal and human subjects
- Assures that subject confidentiality is maintained
- Reviews all university research protocols, funded and unfunded

Sponsored Program Accounting Office (University Budget Office)

- Receives money for a grant project from the funding agency
- Disburses money to pay expenses related to a grant
- Provides periodic budget summaries to grantees
- Makes year-end and financial reports to a funding agency
- Monitors grant expenses

BOX 13.4 *(Continued)*

University Counsel

- Negotiates legal agreements with government and other outside agencies
- Reviews all contracts and agreements with outside agencies
- Protects your rights in disagreements with other scientists or outside agencies
- Oversees complaints about scientific misconduct
- Oversees HIPAA compliance
- Provides oversight to conflict of interest and conflict of commitment policies

As you can see from the descriptions of these offices, universities have a fairly comprehensive infrastructure from which to manage your grant. Since you will be interacting with these offices in both the pre-award and post-award phases of your project, it is important to develop a positive relationship with the professionals in these offices. In light of the increased oversight of grants, it is best that you pay particular attention to three areas in managing your grant. These are managing your budget, following academic policies such as avoiding conflicts of interest, and ensuring that appropriate credit is given to the scholarship that arises from your project.

13.5 BUDGET MANAGEMENT

One very important function of the university's research administration is to oversee the budget of funded grants. After you receive notification of your award, a copy of your approved budget will be sent to the Sponsored Program Accounting Office (SPAO). The SPAO will set up an account for expenses related to your project. This account will be assigned a special number to identify it as a budget for an externally funded project. This is the number that you will use in submitting all grant related expenses within your institution. The budget categories will correspond to those you submitted in your grant proposal. We discussed these budget categories in chapter 6.

In some cases, this budget will be the same as you requested in your grant proposal. In other cases, the agency will have reduced the budget amount by perhaps as much as 20 percent. If there has been a reduction, you will have to consider the changes to your proposed activities that will be necessary to meet the reduced budget. The funding agency may or may not specify the categories from which reductions must be taken. If they do not, then you have to re-compute your budget and provide the SPAO and the funding agency with a revised budget for their approval.

Your institution will have standard forms to use when making purchases or seeking reimbursement for your other grant related expenses. You will need to keep a detailed record of these expenses and ensure that they are reported in the correct budget categories. The SPAO will receive a copy of the various purchase orders and travel reimbursement requests that you submit and keep a running account of the amount of money in each category. They will also automatically deduct the budgeted salaries for all project personnel each month.

As you conduct the project, you must be aware of the expenses that are allowed and those that are not (from OMB Circular A-21). For example, when traveling, you must travel in the most economical way possible. If you fly, that means that you must fly coach and not business or first class, even if there is enough money in the budget category to do so. There is also a federal law that requires that any time you fly, you do so on an American based carrier, even if you can obtain a cheaper fare from a foreign airline. There are some exceptions to this law, so you should either read Circular A-21 or check with your Office of Research Administration. In addition, foreign travel, with the exception of Canada and Mexico, is usually not allowed unless you get permission ahead of time from your Project Officer.

The SPAO will keep track of all of your grant expenses and prepare monthly reports based on receipts from vendors or your travel expenses. However, as we have mentioned before, it is wise to keep your own record of expenses. It is important to monitor these expenses, since there is usually a significant lag time between the date you purchase an item and when it is noted on the monthly reports. Your records will provide a more up-to-date summary of how much you have spent in each category. It is particularly important to have an accurate picture of your budget status at the end of a budget cycle. You will need to know if you have unspent funds, whether the amount of unspent funds exceeds 25% of the total budget for the year, and if you can carry over funds in the next cycle.

Another reason to monitor these reports is that, in busy offices, sometimes expenses from other projects are inadvertently charged to your grant account. If this is the case, you need to contact the Budget Office immediately, since you do not want to find yourself overspent in a category that you need.

13.6 ACADEMIC POLICIES

Another important regulation that you should be aware of is your institution's conflict of interest policy. While not directly related to the management of your grant, you will have to assure your institution and the federal government that the funds you receive to carry out your project do not pose a conflict of interest. In other words, your grant must be carried out to advance the science, rather than to benefit you financially. Potential conflicts of interest can occur in industry-sponsored research, such as drug trials, or those projects that involve technology. For example, if you or a member of your family owned or had significant shares in a company that manufactured assistive devices, it would be a conflict of interest for you to conduct a study that tested the effectiveness of these devices. While policies among universities differ, institutions must assure the federal government that they have a conflict of interest policy in place. As a result, many universities require that all employees sign a statement each year certifying that they do not have significant financial interests in private companies or, if they do, to disclose that interest to the university.

Authorship Policies

Publishing articles based on your research or training grants are usually not required, but they are indeed expected. It is important for you to disseminate the findings of your grant to a wide audience. There are at least five reasons why it is important to disseminate information about your project.

1. The findings from your research or training grant can add to the knowledge base and body of literature in your field.

2. Presentations and publications provide you with more credibility and help you secure future funding.

3. The funding agency likes to see the results of its investment publicized.

4. Dissemination of the results of your project is often a requirement for funding.

5. The number of publications and presentations you do is important to your career since they figure heavily into decisions about promotion, tenure, and future professional opportunities.

Two of the most often used ways to disseminate information is through presentations at scientific meetings and publication in the journals in your field. You may want to involve your investigative team in the dissemination process and begin thinking of appropriate forums relatively soon after you receive notice of funding. Here we focus on guidelines for authorship of publications rather than presentations, however, the same general principles apply to both.

One important consideration in the dissemination process is the way in which you acknowledge the contributions of each person participating in the development of a manuscript. The scientific community needs to know who deserves credit for the work and who is responsible for its scientific integrity. The issue is important enough that many universities, as well as professional and scholarly journals have developed policies that help guide this decision.

There are two considerations that must be addressed in considering authorship of a manuscript. The first is the question of who should qualify as an author. The second is how the level of involvement in the manuscript should be communicated to the scientific community. There is general agreement regarding the first of these considerations. There is little unanimity of opinion regarding the second.

Qualification as an Author

Generally, the criteria for authorship is that anyone listed as an author must have made a significant contribution to the work and be willing and able to take responsibility for its content. This implies such roles as idea conception, study design, analysis, and interpretation of data. It also includes the drafting of the original manuscript and/or critically revising the intellectual content and approval of the version to be published. Being a member of a research group does not automatically give a person the right of authorship. Previously, it was not uncommon for someone to be named as an honorary author because of his/her supervisory position in a laboratory or a research group. However, this practice is no longer acceptable in most scientific journals.

Level of Contribution

There are a number of ways in which the level of a person's contribution is assessed. The most common way to communicate the relative contribution of each author is through the order of names in a manuscript. However, the meaning underlying the order of the authors list does vary significantly across scientific disciplines. In many disciplines or scholarly journals the senior author, or the individual who has the most influence on the manuscript, is listed first and others who contributed are listed in order of the magnitude of their contribution. In some cases, most notably in basic science, the head of a laboratory in which a study is carried out is listed as the last author, whether he or she had any influence in the work. In other disciplines, the senior author is listed last. There is no systematic approach that is accepted by all journals and in all disciplines.

Authorship listing and responsibility should be discussed before a manuscript or presentation is started. Although there is considerable debate about these considerations, the most accepted set of standards, used by over 500 journals in the biomedical and health fields, is called the "Uniform Requirements for Manuscripts Submitted to Medical Journals." The Uniform Requirements recommend that the order of listing be determined beforehand and that the authors and its meaning be stated in the footnote of the manuscript. Given this lack of a systematic approach, many universities in the last decade have developed their own policy or been forced to develop a policy by the federal granting agencies. You should check with the ORA to see if your institution has a written authorship policy.

Box 13.5 presents an example of a policy on authorship used at one university.

BOX 13.5

POLICY ON AUTHORSHIP

Research activity at the University is governed by the tradition of the free exchange of ideas and prompt delivery of research results. The University is committed to the communication of new knowledge to scholars, students, and the public through publication of research results. In order to conform with the Uniform Requirements for Manuscripts Submitted to Biomedical Journals and to ensure the publication of scientific manuscripts which link credit and accountability, the University sets forth this policy on authorship.

Definitions:

Responsible Author (primary author): a person who usually drafts the manuscript, contributes significantly to the published work, and who, together with the Principal Investigator, assumes the public responsibility for the work:

Co-author: a person who has contributed data or made a significant intellectual or practical contribution to the manuscript.

Significant contributor: a person who takes on responsibility for one or more of the following: contribution of experimental data or materials, conception and design, execution or direction of the study, analysis and interpretation of data, and/or preparation or revision of the manuscript.

"Honorary" author: individual who does not satisfy the criteria of authorship by making a significant contribution as defined above to the manuscript.

BOX 13.5 *(Continued)*

Procedure:

An individual who is listed as a responsible author or co-author must make a significant intellectual, technical, or practical contribution as defined above to the project. The concept of "honorary" authorship is prohibited. Such individuals may warrant appropriate acknowledgment in the completed paper.

The responsible author must review the primary data on which the manuscript is based and endorse the conclusions. (S)He must, if requested by sponsors, journals, or federal agencies, provide the data for examination and/or cooperate fully in obtaining and providing the data on which the manuscript is based.

Each co-author must, to the best of his/her ability and within his/her area of expertise, review the manuscript and approve the version to be submitted for publication. (S)He must provide, if requested by sponsors, journals, or Federal agencies, information regarding his/her specific contribution to the manuscript.

As you can see, there are many "hidden" responsibilities associated with a grant award. Most institutions have an infrastructure and knowledge staff to support you in providing appropriate oversight of the award. In this chapter, we have discussed the key requirements you must meet. However, since institutions and each funding agency and/or competition may have other requirements not covered here, it is always best to follow the maxim, "When in doubt, ask."

Bibliography

Blau, P.M. (1964). *Exchange and power in social life.* New York: Wiley.

Brand, M.K., Clark, N., Paavola, F.G., & Pitts, R. (1992). Strengths and weaknesses of allied health special project grant application, *Journal of Allied Health, 21(3)*, 207–218.

DePoy, E., & Gitlin, L. (1998, 2nd Edition). *Introduction to research: Understanding and applying multiple strategies.* St. Louis: Mosby Year Book.

Findley, T.W. (1989). Research in physical medicine and rehabilitation. *American Journal of Physical and Medical Rehabilitation, 68(2)*, 97–102.

Gitlin, L.N., Lyons, K. & Kolodner E. (1994). A model to build collaborative research and education teams. *Educational Gerontology, 20*, 15–34.

Homans, B.C. (1961). *Social behavior: Its elementary forms.* New York: Harcourt, Brace and World.

Jacobs, T.O. (1970). *Leadership and exchange in formal organizations.* Alexandria, VA: Human Resources Research Organization.

Katzenbach, J.R., & Smith, D.K. (1993). The discipline of teams. *Harvard Business Review,* 111–120.

Lyon, S., & Lyon, G. (1980). Team functioning and staff development: A role release approach to providing integrated educational services for severly handicapped students. *Journal of the Association for the Severly Handicapped, 5*, 250–263.

Schumacher, D. (1994). Strategies for helping your faculty get more grants for research. *Research Management Review, 7(1)*, 37–52.

Whitney, F.W. (1990). Passion and collaboration. *Nursing Connections, 3(2)*, 11–15.

Whyte, W.F. (1943). *Street Corner Society.* Chicago: University of Chicago Press.

Appendix A

Common Questions
and their Answers

After reading this book, you may still have questions that are specific to your grant writing situation. Here are 12 questions that individuals commonly ask in our grant writing workshops or while working on a grant application with us, and our responses. We invite other questions you may have after reading this book.

1. *How do I know if a grant is "wired" for a particular institution?*

   First, most competitions sponsored by government agencies and foundations are not wired or earmarked for a particular institution. Occasionally, an agency will publish a call for proposals and/or a contract that is designed for a particular institution with a special area of expertise. This occurs when the agency has a specific focused area or question to solve and a particular institution has both the experience and expertise to address it. However, this situation occurs less often than rumor would have you believe.

   One indication that a competition might be wired is that the eligibility criteria are so specific that they clearly eliminate those without a previous track record or an existing program in the area of the competition. As you network among colleagues who are writing grants, you will quickly learn who has received funding and for what types of projects. This knowledge will increase your understanding of who your competitors might be in a funding competition and whether a particular request for proposals has been developed for a specific institution.

Although a competition may not be wired, it may provide select institutions with a more subtle advantage. For example, in developing a new program area for funding, a program officer in a foundation or federal agency may request the advice and assistance from investigators with a previous record of funding in a similar area. These investigators may be asked to either comment on or suggest a direction for a new program area. A funding announcement that emerges from this process is not wired, but it will obviously reflect the research or educational interests of those who have had input in the process and those funded. This is not to say that other investigators will not be able to develop a competitive application. However, those who have contributed to the development of the new program area will have two advantages. First, they provided input as to the types of projects to be considered for funding and second, they would have had more time to develop a competitive grant. For a more detailed discussion of how funding priorities are developed, see chapter 2 again.

2. *How do you "read between the lines" in a call for proposals?*

There is no easy answer to this question. Reading between the lines is an ability one gains from participating in grantsmanship over the years. The best piece of advice is to read the announcement carefully and ask more experienced colleagues who have had experience with that agency. Learn what journals the agency prefers their funded work to be published in and the language they use to describe the area of inquiry. This will help you identify subtleties in language that will make "reading between the lines" easier.

3. *Why should I bother to submit an application if it is so competitive?*

There is a simple answer to this question. If you do not submit a grant application to a competition that has relevance to your work, we guarantee that you will not be funded. Submitting an application gives you the chance of either being funded or, at the very least, obtaining a critical evaluation of your proposal that can be used to improve your next submission. Keep in mind that few investigators are funded on their first submission. Of course you need to select the competitions that most closely fit your idea and for which you have adequate experience and expertise. In chapter 3, we discuss how to match your level of expertise and interests with funding agencies, while in chapter 9, we discuss different project structures and their relevance for an individual's level of experience.

4. *Are there key "buzz words" I should always use in a grant application?*

You should be able to guess our answer to this question by now. No—there are no magical words or special formulas that can be applied to each grant application, except for the tips, suggestions, and knowledge you have gained by reading the previous chapters. There are key words, however, that may be used by funding agencies to describe either the population of interest or the problem they wish to see addressed. You can learn these terms by reading the description of the funding priority or call for proposals, the professional literature from which the priority has been developed, and by reviewing projects that have been funded in previous competitions.

For example, let's say you plan to submit a grant application to the National Institute on Aging to investigate the role of "caregivers" of individuals with dementia. In the application, terms such as "caregiver," "burden," and "care recipient" could be considered appropriate buzz words since they are clearly defined in the aging literature. However, if you submit an application to the National Institute on Disability and Rehabilitation Research (NIDRR), Department of Education, this agency approaches caregiving from the disability perspective and labels caregivers as "personal care attendants." In writing an application to NIDRR then, a different body of literature as well as terminology would be more appropriate. Chapter 3 discusses how to match your areas of interest and knowledge with a funding agency.

Although there are no hard and fast rules about words to use in all grant applications, we would suggest that you avoid jargon and terminology that is specific to your discipline. While these words are not wrong, they will not strengthen your proposal and, in fact, might weaken it since reviewers may not understand their meaning. We discuss this issue further in chapter 8.

5. *Can I take a project officer to lunch or dinner?*

    The answer to this question is straightforward—NO. Project officers are not permitted to accept gifts. This includes having their lunch, dinner, or participation in an event paid for by a constituent or potential grantee. You may have lunch or dinner with an officer, but may not pick up their tab. Chapter 2 describes the questions you might discuss with a project officer.

6. *Won't a program officer think I'm a nuisance if I call him or her too often?*

    That depends on how often you call and what you call about. It would not be a good strategy to call a program officer once a week, or any time you have a simple question. You should not take their time if you can find an answer to your question elsewhere. However, program officers are public servants, and it is their job to facilitate the submission of high quality projects. As we discussed in chapter 2, it is in the best interests of an agency to obtain as many good proposals as possible. You will also find that many program officers are scientists, well published, and extremely knowledgeable about their own areas of inquiry. They are therefore personally committed to advancing the field and supporting quality and creative proposals.

7. *Do I need an evaluation section in my proposal and, if so, how do I develop one?*

    If you are developing an education or service program, then you will most likely need a plan for its evaluation. There are many excellent books and other resources on program evaluation available, which you can use as a guide. A traditional approach typically involves both formative and summative evaluation strategies. The specific components of your plan will depend upon the objectives of the program and may involve the collection of both qualitative and quantitative information. If you are inexperienced in evaluation, consider adding a consultant to your project or collaborating with individuals in an academic institution who have such expertise. Chapters 9 and 10 discuss the project structures that include a consultative, cooperative or collaborative relationship in more detail.

8. *Do I need to use a model or theory to frame the program I am developing?*

A theory enables an investigator to test a set of principles and explain the outcomes of a research study. Occasionally, a call for proposals will specify that an investigator must explicitly state the theoretical framework on which an intervention or research program is based. An education or service program that is based on a theoretical model will be more competitive than those that are not, since such a program can be replicated and further refined and tested. Review panels recognize that the development of education, service, or research programs grounded in theory or based on testable models are important ways to advance knowledge and practice. Chapter 5 describes the sections of a grant application in more detail and where to introduce and discuss a theoretical framework.

9. *Is it unethical to pay someone, as a consultant, who has served on a review panel to give me advice about my proposal?*

It is not unethical to pay someone to review your proposal. In fact, it is an excellent strategy to improve your work. Individuals who have served on review panels will have an in-depth understanding of the review process and what panel members look for in a proposal. They should also be able to identify "red flags" in your proposal. It is unethical, however, to approach someone who is currently serving on a review panel for a competition in which you have submitted a proposal. Review panel members are ethically bound not to discuss the specific proposals that are submitted.

10. *If I get rejected two or three times, does it mean I should not bother to submit again?*

Not at all. Because of the increasingly competitive nature of the funding environment, it is not uncommon for someone to submit a proposal three or even four times before they are funded. A few years ago, a rule of thumb might have been "three strikes and you're out." This is no longer true. As we discussed in chapter 11, talking to a program officer and carefully reading the reviewers' comments will provide an excellent idea as to whether you should resubmit the proposal. These are better indices of your chances than one or two rejections.

11. *What would you consider the three biggest mistakes that are made in proposals?*

The biggest mistakes made in proposal writing include a failure to read the instructions, disregarding specific topic areas that the application requires to be addressed, or ignoring deadlines.

12. *Do I need a Ph.D. to submit a proposal?*

Legally, you do not. However, a doctoral degree is critical if you plan to be a principal investigator on a research grant since a Ph.D. is considered a research credential. As we have discussed throughout this book, it is very important to demonstrate in the proposal that you have the qualifications to carry out a proposed project. One way to show these qualifications is through your academic credentials. However, another way to present expertise is through a track record of prior research and publication. This is one of the reasons that we have suggested the importance of a professional growth plan (chapter 1) by which to build a history of successful publications and funding. Another strategy to help overcome a lack of credentials would be to work collaboratively with others who have a Ph.D.

Appendix B

Selected Key Acronyms

ACYF	Administration on Children, Youth, and Families
ADA	Americans with Disabilities Act
ADAMHA	Alcohol, Drug Abuse, and Mental Health Administration
ADD	Administration on Developmental Disabilities
AHRQ	Agency for Health Research and Quality (formerly Agency for Health Care Quality and Research)
ANA	Administration for Native Americans
AoA	Administration on Aging
AOTA	American Occupational Therapy Association
AOTF	American Occupational Therapy Foundation
APA	American Psychological Association
APTA	American Physical Therapy Association
BHPr	Bureau of Health Professions
BMCHRD	Bureau of Maternal and Child Health and Resources Development
CBD	Commerce Business Daily
CDBG	Community Development Block Grant
CDC	Centers for Disease Control
CSR	NIH—Center for Scientific Review (formerly the Division of Research Grants)
DADPHP	Division of Associated, Dental, and Public Health Professions
DOC	Department of Commerce
DOD	Department of Defense
DOE	Department of Energy
DOI	Department of Interior
DOJ	Department of Justice

DOL	Department of Labor
DOT	Department of Transportation
FDA	Food and Drug Administration
FIC	Fogarty International Center
FIPSE	Fund for the Improvement of Post-Secondary Education
GAN	Department of Education—Grant Award Notice
HIV	human immunodeficiency virus
HMO	health maintenance organization
HP/DP	health promotion/disease prevention
HRSA	Health Resources and Services Administration
HUD	Department of Housing and Urban Development
IDEA	Individuals with Disabilities Education Act
IHPO	International Health Program Office
IOM	Institute of Medicine of the National Academy of Sciences
IRB	Institutional Review Board
IRG	Integrated Research Group
MCH	maternal and child health
MCHB	Maternal and Child Health Bureau
NCI	National Cancer Institute
NIA	National Institute on Aging
NIAAA	National Institute on Alcohol Abuse and Alcoholism
NIAID	National Institute of Allergy and Infectious Diseases
NIAMS	National Institute of Arthritis and Musculoskeletal and Skin Diseases
NICHD	National Institute of Child Health and Human Development
NIDCD	National Institute on Deafness and Other Communication Disorders
NIDDK	National Institute of Diabetes and Digestive and Kidney Diseases
NIDR	National Institute of Dental Research
NIDRR	National Institute on Disability and Rehabilitation Research
NIH	National Institutes of Health
NIMH	National Institute on Mental Health
NOGA	Notice of Grant Award
NRFC	Not Recommended for Future Consideration
OBRA	Omnibus Budget Reconciliation Act
OHRP	Office for Human Research Protection
OSEP	Office of Special Education Programs
OSERS	Office of Special Education and Rehabilitative Services
OMB	Office of Management and Budget

OMB Circular A-21	Federal "rule book" for university financial arrangements
OMB Circular A-110	Administrative standards for grants and other agreements
OMB Circular A-133	Rules for audits of compliance with federal regulations
PA	Program Announcement
PHS	Public Health Service
RFA	Request for Applications
RFP	Request for Proposals
RO1	Designation for NIH funded Research Projects for independent investigators
R03	NIH—Pilot Research Program
R21	NIH—Exploratory/Development Mechanism
SBIR	NIH—Small Business Innovative Research
SRA	NIH—Scientific Review Administrator
TBI	traumatic brain injury
VA	Department of Veterans Affairs

Appendix C

Select Web Sites

1. List of NIH Institutes: http://www.nih.gov/icd

2. Roster of study sections: http://www.csr.nih.gov/Committees/rosterindex.asp

3. NIH grant review criteria and process: http://www.drg.nih.gov/guidelines/r01.htm

4. NIH peer review http://www.csr.nih.gov/review/policy.asp

5. Department of Education peer review: http://www.ed.gov/pubs/peerreview/execsumm.html

6. Catalog of Domestic Assistance: http://www.cfda.gov

7. Federal Register: http://www.gpo.gov/su_docs/aces/aces140.html

8. Commerce Business Daily: http://www.fedbizopps.gov/—or http://www.cbd.cos.com

9. Federal Rule Book—OMB Circular A-21: http://www.whitehouse.gov/omb/circulars/a021/a021.html

10. Federal administrative standards for administering grants—OMB Circular A-110: http://www.whitehouse.gov/omb/circulars/a110/a110.html

11. Federal rules for audits of compliance with federal regulations—OMB Circular A-133: http://www.whitehouse.gov/omb/circulars/a133/a133.html

12. NIH Grants Policy: http://www.grants.nih.gov/grants/policy/nihgps_2001

13. National Science Foundation Grants Policy Manual: http://www.nsf.gov/pubs/stis1995/nsf9526/nsf9526.txt

14. Health People 2010: http://www.healthypeople.gov/

15. NIH guide (electronic availability): http://grants/nih/gov/grants/guide/

16. NIH modular budgeting: http://grants.nih.gov/grants/funding/modular/modular.htm

Appendix D

Sample Time Line, Budget Sheets, and Flow Charts

SAMPLE TIME LINE

OBJECTIVES	COMPONENT/ACTIVITY	Yr. 1 Fall	Yr. 1 Spring	Yr. 1 Summer	Yr. 2	Yr. 3	Team Leader(s) of Activity
1. Increase the number of allied health professionals working with underserved populations.	a. Students work with faculty mentors to develop strategies to work in medically underserved areas.		X	X	X	X	CD & FP
	b. Design and implement an online network of health promotion consultants on the health promotion website.		X	X	X	X	CD & FP
	c. Recruit program graduates to serve as health promotion consultants.				X	X	CD
2. Expand the knowledge and skills of faculty to design and teach an interdisciplinary community health promotion curriculum using interactive health communication skills.	a. Faculty conduct a comprehensive literature search on interactive health communication curricula and evaluate the top 20 health promotion web-sites to determine applications that are appropriate for individuals with disabilities.	X	X	X			CD
	b. Plan and implement a series of knowledge building meetings for the faculty.	X	X	X	X	X	CD
	c. Faculty work closely with the web design expert to design Interactive Health Communication course.						CD & WC

Key: Team Management Structure
Director (D); Co-Directors (CD); Research Coordinator (RC); Web Design Consultant (WC); OT-PT Fieldwork Preceptor (FP); Advisory Board (AB)

SAMPLE BUDGET WORK SHEET
EDUCTIONAL PROJECT

Personnel   Time/Effort   Dollar Amount Requested

Name	Title	%	Hours/Week	Salary	Fringe	Total
Name #1	Project Director					
Name #2	Project Coordinator					
Name #3	Clinical Coordinator					
Name #4	Academic Coordinator					
Name #5	Project Evaluator					
Name #6	Project Secretary					

Subtotals

Consultant Costs	
Equipment (itemize)	
Contracts	
Supplies (itemize by category)	
Staff Travel	
Other expenses	

Other Expenses

Subtotals

Total Direct Costs

FIGURE 1   Research Design

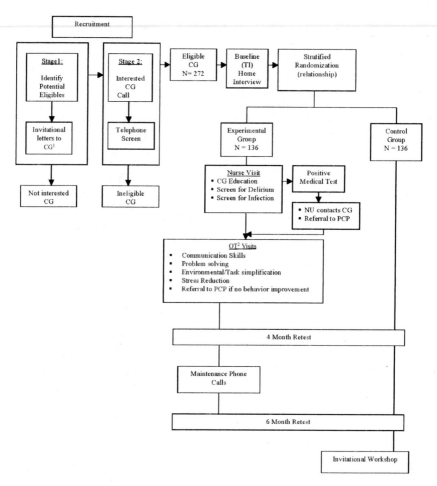

[1] CG = Caregivers
[2] OT = Occupational Therapist

FIGURE 2   Flow Chart of Education Project

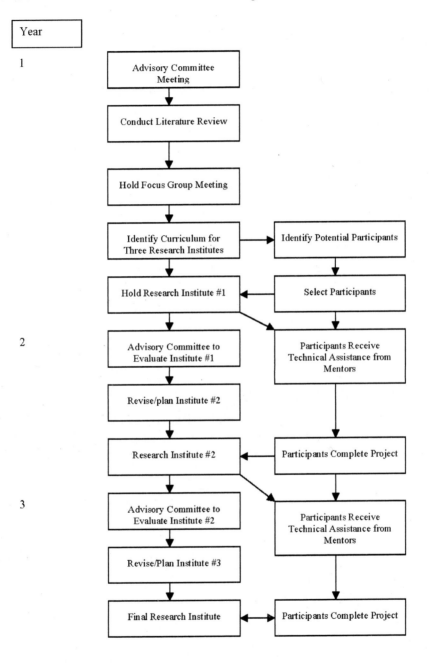

Appendix E

Guidelines for Evaluating Collaborative Teams

CHARACTERISTICS OF COLLABORATION

1. Clear statement of goals, expectations, and procedures

    a. Are members of the project team aware of the goals of the project?

    b. Do all members of the team fully accept the goals of the group?

    c. Does each member of the team understand his/her individual responsibilities?

    d. Does each member of the team understand the procedures that must be followed to complete the project?

2. Role Differentiation

    a. Does each member of the team have specified roles and responsibilities?

    b. Do team members feel responsible for accomplishing the goals of the project?

3. Open Communication

    a. Do members listen and pay attention to what other team members have to say?

    b. Are the ideas and feelings of all members expressed openly and honestly?

4. Open, Honest Negotiation

    a. Do team members feel free to suggest ideas for the direction of a project?

    b. Are differences of opinion sought out and clarified?

    c. Do team members feel free to disagree openly with each other's ideas?

5. Mutual Goals

    a. Are team members committed to carrying out the group's task as opposed to advancing their own interests?

    b. Are goals established by means of group participation?

    c. Are these goals and procedures accepted by each member of the team?

6. Climate of Trust

   a. Do team members feel free to describe their ideas, feelings, and reactions to what is taking place in the group?

   b. other members disclose their ideas, feelings, and reactions to what is currently taking place in the group?

   c. Do team members have respect, confidence, and trust in one another?

   d. Do members of the team engage in extensive and friendly interaction with one another?

7. Cooperation

   a. Do team members seek out opportunities to work with one another on tasks?

   b. Do team members take turns volunteering for specific tasks?

8. Shared Decision Making

   a. Do team members take responsibility for providing input into group decisions?

   b. Do team members have significant input into group decisions for which they have expertise?

9. Conflict Resolution

   a. Are disagreements brought out into the open and faced directly?

   b. When disagreements arise, do members speak freely and openly about their positions?

   c. Do members of the team feel free to disagree with others about procedures or ideas?

   d. Do team members strive to ensure that they do not change their mind about an issue just to avoid conflict and reach agreement and harmony?

10. Equality of Participation

    a. Does each individual, in light of his/her experience and skills, feel free to provide input to team deliberations?

    b. Is discussion distributed among all team members rather than dominated by any one perspective or person?

    c. Are the opinions of members of the teams valued by other members?

11. Group Cohesion

    a. Do members try to make sure others enjoy being members of the team?

    b. Do team members express acceptance and support when other members disclose their ideas, feelings, and reactions to what is currently taking place in the group?

    c. Do team members try to make other members feel valued and appreciated?

    d. Do team members include other members in group activities?

12. Decision by Consensus

    a. Do team members listen to and consider other members' points of view before pressing their ideas?

    b. When discussion reaches a stalemate, do team members look for the next most acceptable alternative?

    c. Do team members avoid engaging in techniques such as majority rule, voting, and coin tossing to reach a decision?

    d. Does the team make sure everybody accepts a solution to a problem for similar reasons?

13. Shared Leadership

    a. Do members of the team assume responsibility for making decisions for the group related to task accomplishment?

    b. Does the formal team leader facilitate discussion rather than dominate it?

    c. Are members of the team given formal responsibility for guiding the group to accomplish certain tasks?

14. Shared Responsibility for Participation

    a. Do all members of the team participate in discussions about important issues?

QUESTIONNAIRE ON COLLABORATION:
INDIVIDUAL ROLE

The following questions are designed to gather information about your participation on [your current] project. Please respond to each honestly using the following scale.

1 = not at all   *2 = somewhat*   *3 = moderately*   *4 = very*

TO WHAT EXTENT:

1. Are you familiar with the goals of this project?

   1   2   3   4

2. Do you endorse the goals of this project?

   1   2   3   4

3. Do you feel responsible for carrying out the goals of this project?

   1   2   3   4

4. Have you been assigned specific responsibilities to carry out the project?

   1   2   3   4

5. Do you understand what is expected of you?

   1   2   3   4

6. Do you understand the procedures necessary to complete the project?

   1   2   3   4

7. Do you listen to what other team members have to say?

   1   2   3   4

8. Do you feel free to express your feelings about an issue in the group?

   1   2   3   4

9. Do you express your feelings honestly about an issue in the group?

   1   2   3   4

10. Do you feel free to suggest ideas about the direction of the project?

   1   2   3   4

11. Do you feel free to disagree with other group members?

   1   2   3   4

12. Do you provide support to others when they make their ideas, feelings or reactions known?

   1   2   3   4

13. Do you have confidence in other group members?

   1   2   3   4

14. Do you volunteer for specific group tasks?

   1   2   3   4

15. Do you take responsibility to provide your expertise in group decisions?

   1   2   3   4

16. Do you value the opinions of other group members?

   1   2   3   4

17. Are you willing to assume responsibility for making a decision for the group in areas where you have expertise?

   1   2   3   4

18. Do you try to participate in group discussions?

   1   2   3   4

19. Do you feel a real part of the team?

   1   2   3   4

20. Do you feel comfortable when differences of opinion are expressed or there is conflict?

   1   2   3   4

Please circle one:

   Member of Faculty   Community Member

   Other Faculty   Clinician

QUESTIONNAIRE ON COLLABORATION:
EVALUATION OF GROUP FUNCTIONING

The following questions are designed to gather information about the participation of other members of your group on [your current] project. Please respond to each honestly using the following scale. Try to think of the group as a whole. So, if some members behave in certain ways and other members do not, then respond to the question somewhere in the middle of the scale.

1 = not at all   *2 = somewhat*   *3 = moderately*   *4 = very*

TO WHAT EXTENT DO YOU BELIEVE OTHER MEMBERS:

1. Are familiar with the goals of this project?

   1   2   3   4

2. Accept the goals of this project?

   1   2   3   4

3. Feel responsible for carrying out the goals of this project?

   1   2   3   4

4. Have been assigned specific responsibilities to carry out the project?

   1   2   3   4

5. Understand what is expected of them?

   1   2   3   4

6. Understand the procedures necessary to complete the project?

   1   2   3   4

7. Listen to what other team members have to say?

   1   2   3   4

8. Feel free to express their feelings about an issue in the group?

   1   2   3   4

9. Express their feelings honestly about an issue in the group?

   1   2   3   4

10. Feel free to suggest ideas about the direction of the project?

   1   2   3   4

11. Feel free to disagree with each other about an idea?

     1   2   3   4

12. Offer support when other members make their ideas, feelings or reactions known?

     1   2   3   4

13. Have confidence that other group members will complete assigned tasks?

     1   2   3   4

14. Volunteer for specific group tasks?

     1   2   3   4

15. Take responsibility for providing their expertise in group decisions?

     1   2   3   4

16. Value the opinions of other group members?

     1   2   3   4

17. Are willing to assume responsibility for making a decision for the group in areas where they have expertise?

     1   2   3   4

18. Participate in the group discussion?

     1   2   3   4

19. Look at the tasks of the team?

     1   2   3   4

20. Feel a real part of the team?

     1   2   3   4

21. Feel comfortable when differences of opinion are expressed or there is conflict?

     1   2   3   4

Please circle one:

    Member of Faculty   Community Member

    Other Faculty   Clinician

Index